D0729433

Juli and Jessica Dixon give a compelling personal account of a family fighting for its sanity, its wholeness, and its sense of normal during an unplanned journey. Be prepared to cry, to cheer, to hope, and to be amazed.

—**Timothy D. Kanold, Ph.D.**, former superintendent of Adlai E. Stevenson High School District 125, a recurring recipient of the Blue Ribbon School Award of Excellence by the United States Department of Education.

Juli and Jessica recount their family's heartbreaking struggle and triumph, teaching us the healing power of optimism, love, and determination. Though humbled by their anguish, we're inspired by their defining choices of hope over sorrow and action over complacency. Alex's journey is a cherished lesson to every reader.

—**Eric A. Sheldon, M.D.**, Founder and Medical Director, Miami Research Associates

As a special education professor, this book brought home the numerous issues that are created, impacted, and exacerbated by a disability. Alex's story helps us value life, widen our perspective, and open our hearts.

—**Wendy W. Murawski, Ph.D.**, Executive Director of the Center for Teaching & Learning at California State University, Northridge; author of *Collaborate, Communicate, & Differentiate!;* and President of the Teacher Education Division of the Council for Exceptional Children

For
ALEX

*"Remember that sometimes
not getting what you want
is a wonderful stroke of luck."*

—His Holiness, the 14th Dalai Lama

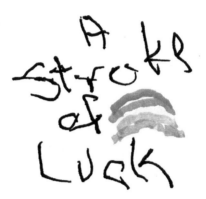

A Stroke of Luck

Thank you for all that
you do to help others.

Keep smiling !!

Alex Dixon

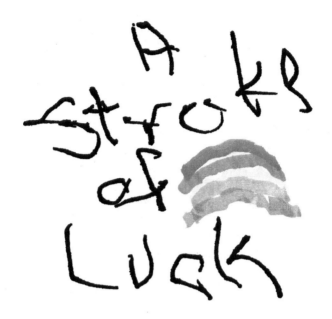

A Girl's Second Chance at Life

Juli K. Dixon, Ph.D. with Jessica Dixon

Finding Words Press

A Stroke of Luck: A Girl's Second Chance at Life

Copyright © 2013 by Juli K. Dixon and Jessica Dixon. Finding Words Press. All Rights Reserved.

No part of this publication may be reproduced, stored in a retrieval system or transmitted, in any form or by any means—electronic, mechanical, photocopying, recording or otherwise—without prior written permission from the publisher, except for the inclusion of brief quotations in a review.

Some names and identifying details have been changed to protect the privacy of individuals.

For information about this title or to order other books and/or electronic media, contact the publisher:

Finding Words Press
www.astrokeofluck.net
www.julidixon.com

ISBN:
978-0-9898088-0-4 paperback
978-0-9898088-1-1 hardcover
978-0-9898088-2-8 e-book

Cover design: Jordan Barrett
Printed in the United States of America
First Edition

Table of Contents

Challenge is challenge and life is life,
but something between them just doesn't seem
right.

Sometimes you hear that heartwarming song
and sometimes you hear nothing at all

but challenge is challenge and life is life,
and something between them just doesn't seem
right.

Sometimes life's a gift and sometimes I can't tell,
sometimes it's love and sometimes it's hell.

Sometimes it's laughter and sometimes it's fate;
all I know is that it's not always great.

I have been through a lot. I have seen everything.
But most of all I want to feel good again.

Challenge is challenge and life is life,
but something between them just doesn't
seem right.

—By Alex Dixon (age 10)
in an email to her mother on April 10, 2008

PART I: SUDDEN ILLNESS

1

An Unreal Journey

Alex was a normal, healthy, bright girl. Other than a series of minor fractures from skateboarding, jumping off a swing, or catching a football, she had no health issues. She loved to play outside on the swings and in the fort connected to the swing set with her little sister, Jessica. They made mud pies when it rained and villages for their Littlest Pet Shop animals on dry days. Alex enjoyed swimming, horseback riding, and sailing with her family. She drew beautiful pictures and took many art classes. She loved animals so much that she planned to be a veterinarian when she grew up. Alex played the piano, and had taken lessons since she was six.

On January 27, 2008, she participated in her first piano competition. She came home from the competition with a fever, a severe headache, and lower back pain. She curled up on the couch and was not able to completely straighten out her body again for over two years.

The Beginning of a Very Long Illness

"Don't!"

I can't believe that Alex doesn't even want me to rub her back. She always wants her back rubbed. She is just like Marc;

she can just lie there for hours if someone is rubbing her back. I can't sit still that long. Now she's been lying here on the couch for three days without wanting anyone to touch her. When she walks to the bathroom, she can't even stand all the way up; she sort of just hobbles. I think it is time to take her to see the doctor. She has had a high fever and headache for long enough and I don't understand why her lower back hurts her so much. She describes it as pain pinging back and forth between two points in her back. It is just weird.

"I'm taking you to see Dr. Conway." I feel so fortunate to be close friends with the girls' pediatrician. I try not to abuse the friendship. It even feels natural to call her "Dr. Conway" when we discuss medical things and "Alex" when we don't. Our relationship works. We rarely get to spend time together because of the crazy-long hours we both put into our jobs, but when we do connect, we are like sisters.

Dr. Conway doesn't know what to make of Alex either. She examines Alex for a long time and eventually sends us to the emergency room. We drive straight from Dr. Conway's office to the children's hospital. I guess I wasn't overreacting by bringing Alex in to the doctor.

I hate emergency rooms. I don't like thinking about all the germs and things you can catch from other people. I don't like to touch anything or have my children touch anything. Having to go through a metal detector to enter this ER doesn't make me feel any better.

We wait for what seems like forever to get called back. I suppose that is a good sign; when you get called back right away you know you are the worst case. The first thing the ER doctors do is to take an x-ray of Alex's chest. I don't know why—she isn't coughing. She doesn't even have a cold. I suppose we will wait for another hour or so to find out that it is normal. At least we are in our own little room in the emergency area. We have our door closed and Alex is watching the Disney Channel on a little TV while I am trying to keep from calling people. When I am nervous, I call people. I guess I'm nervous. I didn't expect Dr. Conway to send us to the emergency room. That threw me for a loop. I want to call my mom and Valerie, my sister-in-law, to tell them what is going on but I don't want to alarm Alex. It is better that she is watching TV. I find myself drawn into a rerun as well.

"Mom, can I see you for a moment?"

Why does the doctor want to see me in the hall? This can't be good.

"Mom, we found what looks like a mass in Alex's lung. We would like to take her in for a CT scan as soon as possible. I've ordered it stat so we should be able to get her in right away."

"What are you talking about? She's not complaining of pain in her chest, just in her back."

"We'll know more after the CT scan. You can go with her."

They take her right away; I don't even have time to call Marc or my mom. I can barely breathe during the entire procedure. The doctor tells me that the CT scan is needed to rule out cancer. Cancer!

They rule out cancer, thank God. But they rule in pneumonia. This just doesn't make sense. Alex has no symptoms of pneumonia; she has no cough, no cold, no shortness of breath. And yet, she has severe pneumonia in the upper lobe of her left lung and persistent pain in two focal points in her lower back on the right side. What is the connection?

They admit her to the hospital in Orlando. She has another CT scan, bone scans, MRIs, x-rays, and blood tests over the course of five days. Doctors treat her for resistant pneumonia with heavy-duty antibiotics. Alex is ten. She has unfortunately never learned to swallow pills. The only option is to give her an absolutely awful-tasting liquid antibiotic we name the vomit drug. The only way she can get it down is to chew up a bit of chocolate, leave it in her mouth, then try to gulp down the medicine cup of liquid. Her face twists in a way that you just know she tastes something unimaginably bad. Then she quickly chews the rest of the piece of chocolate so she won't gag and vomit the medicine. I don't even dare taste the antibiotic but Marc sticks his finger in the remains of the medicine cup and tastes it. He says it really is the worst thing he has ever tasted. Alex toughs it out and completes the antibiotic. Her pneumonia resolves, but the lower back pain persists. Alex is sort of whiny. Every time the doctors come by and ask her how she is feeling, she tells them that she feels terrible. Even as her pneumonia resolves, she continues to say she feels terrible. We are sent home with the attending pediatrician fairly sure that Alex is using her symptoms for attention and she is actually fine. They can't identify any other reason for her to still be acting this way.

Alex spends the next several weeks at home curled up on the couch, not well enough to go to school and in too much pain. Things are rough in the Dixon household.

"Alex, you have to eat. It is not a choice."

She always has an appetite. She eats the healthiest of all the children I know. Her favorite foods are spinach and black beans and rice. She can pack it away. How can she be refusing to eat now? Is she just doing it for attention like the doctors said? Well, she will just have to sit at the table until she eats. I don't care how long it takes. I have made her everything she likes and now it is up to her.

"I'm not hungry, I just want to go to my room." Alex eats the very minimum she can get away with and then gets up to go to her room. She is walking so poorly. She isn't straightening her right leg all the way and she is not putting her heel down to the floor. She is bent over like an old woman. She doesn't seem to be willing to put her weight on her right leg as she slowly makes her way to her room. She seems to prefer being alone in her room more than being out with the family. That is unusual as Alex is not a loner. She prefers to be around family at all times. She even prefers to share a room with her sister rather than live in her own space. We lived in a townhouse for a few months and the girls had to share a room. When we moved into a larger house, Alex did not want to have her own room. Not anymore. Now she wants to close herself up in her room all alone. This is one unhappy child.

Wednesday, February 27, 2008

Dear Diary,

Me again! My parents act like nothing is going on when I am in my room crying. I bet they don't know! They don't really care very much! I hate hurting and feeling upset and not sleeping and feeling sick at the same time! HELP!!!! I am going to record my feelings so it will never happen again! It is hard being me! I know that I am lucky but still!

—*Alex*

P.S. I feel like a smushed bug on a windshield but way off where the wiper can't reach!

We have to get to the bottom of this. Someone just has to have answers. We begin to see a long string of specialists: rheumatologists, orthopedists, neurologists, anesthesiologists, geneticists, and the list goes on.

Alex

Alex was a beautiful baby. The type you see in commercials with thick, curly, dark brown hair and big brown eyes like almonds. She was a happy baby too. She passed all her milestones early. Once she started talking she didn't stop. When she was five years old, she was interviewed for a video to market her preschool. The director for the video asked the teacher if there was a preschooler who might be comfortable talking on camera. The teacher immediately suggested Alex. The director asked Alex what she wanted to be when she grew up and she told him she wanted to be a farmer. She went on and on about how she had a chicken named April at a petting farm (we neglected to tell her that every time we went to this petting farm she would identify a new chicken as April and think it was the original chicken she had befriended and named as her pet). She also said that she knew how to milk a cow. She had the director and the entire video crew in hysterics. Adults would say that they felt like they were talking to another adult when conversing with Alex. She was six going on twenty-six, seven going on twenty-seven, and so on. She perceived beyond her years from an early age. That may be why she always seemed to become the teacher's pet.

She also developed a dry sense of humor. She was quite intelligent and understood the nuances of sarcasm. She was great to be around. We had a wonderfully open relationship and I valued the time we spent together. Her conversations were interesting and she was quite engaging. She saw a psychologist for some anxiety issues at one point. Our challenge was finding a psychologist who could meet her on her level. One psychologist we tried had an office in a one-story building with beautiful oak trees that were strung with hanging Spanish moss. The trees were clearly visible through the window in her office. Alex's visits to psychologists would begin with me meeting with the psychologist while Alex waited in the waiting area and then we would switch places. The entire time I sat with this particular psychologist I found my eyes wandering away from her face and toward the large window high on the wall to one of the trees, a great big tree with low-hanging thick branches. The distraction was almost to the point where I had a difficult time focusing on her questions. Coincidentally, according to Alex, this psychologist's strategy for helping her to cope with anxiety was to imagine a tree and take her worries and pin them on the worry tree. That way she would not have to carry her worries with her through life—they could be left on the worry tree. Alex went along with the doctor for the entire session. When the session was finished, Alex told me that she could not go back. She said that she didn't want to hurt the psychologist's feelings but really it was the psychologist who needed help, because how was some made-up tree in her mind going to solve her problems? For some time after, whenever things were tough, Alex would say, "Now where is that worry tree when I need it?" I would visualize the tree outside the psychologist's office. I wonder if Alex did the same. I never asked her. We would both laugh and things would seem better.

Alex was a high achiever in academics. She read early and enjoyed writing. She entered the gifted program in primary school. Eligibility was determined by an IQ test. She scored well. She was not athletic, however. Her cousins were cheerleaders and soccer players. At family events they would run and play catch. Alex would run with them but she sort of stumble ran, and she was quite slow. Catching a ball was also a challenge. When we finally taught her to catch a football she broke her finger the very same day. She did not have a desire to participate in team sports, instead preferring art and science camps and music lessons. She did enjoy sailing, skiing, and horseback riding but those didn't require the same level of physical prowess. Busy and happy in her activities, she didn't seem to notice her lack of ability.

She could talk to anyone about anything as long as the person wasn't her peer. Her greatest challenge came in interacting with peers. She just didn't know what to say to them. She felt uncomfortable and became quite negative. We described her as seeing the cup as half empty rather than half full. We prepared her to enter social situations so that she would not stay in the background. She really struggled socially through much of elementary school. We used to say that she did not need school for the academics but rather for the social experiences it provided. In first grade, when I arrived at school to pick her up from the extended day program, I saw most of the children playing in the playground. They were running around but she hung back from the others, not sure how to engage in their play. Shortly after that I hired a babysitter to pick her up from school so she didn't have to go to the extended day program. She was happy to invite one child from the neighborhood to come to play after school.

She had friends but not many. Typically they were like herself, bright kids who didn't quite fit the mold. Second and third grades were tough. By fourth grade she finally began to feel comfortable with a group of friends. They invited her to their homes and she enjoyed going. She began letting herself loose with them. She was invited to a birthday party that involved kids' makeovers. The girls were made to look like pop stars. They even put on a show for the parents as we picked them up at the end of the party. Alex came home looking like Hannah Montana—wig and all.

This was why we were so surprised by her change in attitude when she got sick. She had finally become happy in all sorts of situations before she got sick. After she got sick she became anything but happy. Her beautiful face took on a mask of pain. It didn't make sense for her to act this way now; she didn't need the extra attention—things were going well. What had caused the change?

2

Searching for Answers

I call Dr. Conway for advice. "Alex doesn't seem to be getting better. She doesn't want to eat; she doesn't want to leave her room. She is miserable. She says she is still in pain. She won't do anything. The muscles in her right leg seem to be getting tighter and tighter."

"It might be time to see a psychiatrist. It sounds like she is truly depressed. I have heard good things about Dr. Franklin." Dr. Conway knows that we need a smart psychiatrist to work with Alex. Someone who will approach her on her level—no worry trees. Dr. Conway thinks that it might be possible that her muscles are getting tighter because she won't get up and move around. Could this be from depression?

We bring Alex to a psychiatrist who meets with Marc and me while Alex waits in the waiting room. She just lies down on the couch and waits. She doesn't even mind staying there alone. After we are done sharing our thoughts about Alex, he meets with her. Alex doesn't like him.

"He's stupid. All he had me do was draw pictures. How is that going to help me get better?"

"You have to trust him. Dr. Conway says he is smart and I agree. He's an M.D. and a Ph.D. He says that taking Prozac should help because it helps with pain and depression. You seem to have both." She recovered from the pneumonia almost two months ago. Maybe it *is* depression. Regardless, the Prozac should help. At least it can't hurt—or so we think. We fill the prescription and never see the doctor again.

Shortly after Alex begins taking Prozac she gets angry. She yells at everyone about everything. She even yells at her dog, Buttons, and she loves him more than anything. The two of them are connected. Before Alex got sick she would play outside with Jessica and their friend Josh. If they didn't take Buttons, he would pace and whimper the entire time she was gone. He would let her do anything to him—even dress him up in the Hannah Montana wig from that birthday party.

Alex says that she feels like she can't control her anger. Marc and I don't know what to do about it. We finally send her back to school after being out for almost two months; she needs to make up her fourth-grade state exams. She doesn't want to go. She stays angry while she is at school but manages to hold in her temper until the car ride home. I pick her up and she lets loose.

"Mom, you shouldn't have made me go to school. You're ass!"

"Alex, if you're going to swear, you should at least swear with proper grammar. It isn't 'you're ass,' it's 'you're an ass.'" Well, that leaves her speechless but holy cow, swearing? Alex doesn't swear. I'm so glad I didn't yell back at her. One for mom . . . but seriously, this is just wrong. She really is angry and acting out of character. What monster has taken over my daughter? I need to get her back in to the psychiatrist. I don't think this medicine is working.

I call her psychiatrist and ask if the drug can actually change her personality. He brushes me off and tells me he can't see us for a month.

Alex's anger intensifies quickly. Within the week she becomes unsafe. We contact a psychologist she had seen the previous year after the worry-tree incident. He lives and practices in Gainesville, Florida, over two hours from our home. He says it sounds like she is having a textbook reaction to the Prozac but he needs to see her to be sure. He tells us how to slowly take her off the Prozac. By this time, she has threatened Jessica and Buttons. Jessica is only seven years old.

"We have to get Jessica and Buttons out of the house. It just isn't safe. I'm going to the neighbors to see if Jessica can go there. I will put the dog outside in a crate and ask Suzanne to pick him up." Marc is taking this seriously. He calls Suzanne, the lady from whom we adopted Buttons two years earlier, and brings Jessica next door. I call my mother and ask her to come get Jessica from the neighbors' and bring her back to my mom's house. She is at home so it takes her a little more than an hour to get here.

"Alex, you have to stop pushing and hitting us." I've got my arms around her but it isn't enough. It seems like she wants me to hold her but she is like a caged animal. She doesn't even sound human. She is moaning, grunting, screaming, and crying. She is wild and destructive, even her eyes look wild—wide open and darting all around. She breaks free and starts grabbing toys off her shelves and throwing them. Her room is no longer safe for her.

"Jules, we have to clear her things out of her room. She's going to destroy everything and hurt herself." Marc begins to empty the contents of Alex's room through the Jack-and-Jill bathroom into Jessica's room, taking breakable objects like picture frames first. I'm glad her room is carpeted.

"Alex, let me hold you; come here." I am attempting unsuccessfully to serve as a sort of human straightjacket. She continues to grab at anything she can. She takes a book and starts tearing it in pieces. She loves books and the one she has in her hands is her favorite. She is making a strange noise, sort of moaning. This is scary. There is nothing left in her room now but her furniture and some books. At least she will be safe as long as we stay with her.

She stands up and pulls over her bookcase. Marc and I manage to keep it from hurting her and us. I don't know where her strength comes from after two months of lying around barely walking. It reminds me of a time when I was in high school at an extracurricular event. One of the students took some sort of drug—I have no idea what as I was not part of that crowd. He went crazy. He jumped off a high stage like it was nothing. He climbed a tall fence, looking almost superhuman. An ambulance finally had to come for him. I was scared then as a teenager. I am much more frightened now as a parent. What is happening to Alex? We take all of her furniture from her room other than her mattress. There are torn pages from the books we left with her scattered all over the floor. We decide to leave them because she seems to need something destructive to do with her hands. My parents keep calling but we can't talk. They are left in the dark—they'll have to wait to find out what is going on—their only information coming from Jessica. I can't even imagine what she is making of this situation.

Marc and I are using everything we have in us to keep Alex safe. She cannot be alone. Marc and I are basically a tag team. We can't keep this up. I call my friend and colleague, Lisa, to come help. She is a professor of special education. She will know what to do. She comes immediately and joins our team. Marc and I finally have a few minutes to talk out a plan. We need to make it through the night and now that Lisa is here we can do this. Based on the psychologist's suggestion, we will give Alex a few Benadryl in the morning, wait for her to get sleepy, and then drive her to Gainesville to see him.

The night is rough. Alex has never been violent like this before. She hits us and yells awful things. She does the same thing to Lisa. Lisa is amazing. She stays cool while Alex is absolutely out of control. We are so frightened. We give her the Benadryl in the morning, put her in the car, and drive to Gainesville. The psychologist says that it is as he suspected, Alex is experiencing a textbook reaction to Prozac. It is not an allergy but an undesirable response connected to the drug's use. She cannot control her behavior. We have to just continue to keep her (and us) safe while the drug works its way out of her system. We can't just stop the medication; we have to taper her off of it instead. I hate to have to keep giving her something that has this effect on her. There is talk of admitting her to a hospital psych ward. No way. Marc and I decide to keep her with us and wait out the diminishing effects of the drug. We go to a hotel room in Gainesville. She screams and fights but slowly becomes less destructive. I wonder what people who are staying in the rooms that surround ours must think—not that it matters. We didn't choose this either.

How could the prescribing psychiatrist have let us down so badly? He should have responded when I called him with my concerns. Alex became his responsibility along with ours as soon as he prescribed medication for her. It was just plain irresponsible of him to push us off when we needed him. He is to become one of many specialists who let Alex down.

"Tricking" Alex

By now we are in a panic. What's going on? Could this be part of some sort of anxiety? Is there some disease we're missing? Why isn't she better? The pneumonia is gone but our Alex isn't back.

We decide it is time for a pediatric neurologist. Her pediatrician supports this and helps us get an appointment quickly—this is no small feat. We go to the neurologist and things just seem to get more surreal. Over the next several visits the neurologist assesses Alex using a series of tests, some of which are quite painful. The results are all negative and yet Alex is still in pain, she cannot straighten her leg all the way, and she walks with an abnormal gait.

The neurologist is running out of ideas and questions Alex's integrity. On one visit—the last visit—the doctor meets Alex at the entrance to the examining room hallway. He says, "Hi, Alex!" a little too brightly and puts his arm around her shoulder. I am still in the process of gathering our belongings from the waiting room, so I am trailing behind. The next thing I see is the doctor begin to jog down the hall with his arm around Alex, who is tripping over herself and falling to the carpeted hallway floor. I don't even run to her immediately. I am dumbfounded, frozen in place. I just witnessed a neurologist drag my daughter down the hall . . . . He was trying to trick her into running! He hoped to catch her off guard so she would return to a normal gait. Alex falls down. She feels so confused by his behavior but this does not convince the neurologist. He accuses Alex of malingering to get more attention from me because I work too much and travel too much for my work.

I know it is ludicrous, but at the same time "mother's guilt" creeps in. Maybe I do work too much. As a mathematics education professor at a university, I travel to present at conferences or work on national committees several times per year. I also travel to work with school districts throughout the country. I have always traveled. I thought my children were used to it. Would she have gotten sick like this if I had been home more?

She always wants me to spend more time with her. I do spend quite a bit of time with her but she always seems to want more. Could she be vying for my attention? Even if she is, could this illness really be a by-product? It just doesn't make sense. Alex does focus on her illness. She sometimes even exaggerates her symptoms so that the doctors can see what is wrong and will know she is really sick. This clearly works to her disadvantage. I try to explain this to her many times. At ten years old, to her it is the only way to get help, to let the doctors see she needs help. It isn't on purpose. I don't think she even realizes she is doing it until I point it out. When I can't change Alex's behavior, I try to change the doctors' perceptions. They are the educated adults. You would hope that they could see through Alex's barriers to her needs. This does not prove to be the case. It makes a bad situation worse—certainly with this neurologist.

We are running out of options. Alex's leg won't straighten and she suffers with severe pain. We shift our energy to working with a physical therapist to try to resolve her leg issue. It has been two months since Alex got sick.

Stretching Beyond Alex's Limit

In March 2008, Alex begins intensive physical therapy at a hospital in Orlando. She works with a physical therapist three times per week for an hour per session. Her groin is very tight. Therapy focuses on stretching her groin and straightening and strengthening her leg. We support these efforts with home exercises as well. Alex does not appear motivated. She is compliant but not motivated. She agrees to sleep in all sorts of contraptions to stretch her leg and groin. One brace separates her legs and doesn't allow her to move. She says she feels like a turtle stuck on its back. She can't even get up at night to use the bathroom without calling Marc or me to get her out of her brace first and then put it back on after she is done. She doesn't complain but she also doesn't seem to try as hard as she can. She doesn't make much improvement. Marc and I push her and push her without results. We do every single home exercise the physical therapist prescribes. We never miss a night. We yell so much. We yell at each other for being too hard or too easy, or sometimes even both. We yell at each other to stop yelling. We yell at Alex to work harder, to stretch more, to do whatever it takes to straighten her leg. Alex yells back at us that we just don't understand. She yells that she is doing the best she can. It is difficult to keep from doubting Alex. I guess we are guilty of behaving like the doctors who don't trust her. If we can't figure out what is wrong, and we can't help Alex, maybe nothing is wrong. Maybe she is doing this for attention. Marc and I fight an inner war. At least we think it is inner. It isn't. Alex knows how we feel.

I certainly spend a tremendous amount of time with Alex, taking her to therapy, working with her at home, and discussing her situation. Could she be making herself sick to spend more time with me? These awful thoughts creep into my mind when I try to sleep, when I drive, even when I'm working with Alex. The same thing happens to Marc. In weak moments we say awful things to Alex, such as, "Are you doing this because you want to be sick?" and "Are you doing this for attention?" We speak out of frustration and fear; we believe her and believe in her more than we doubt—but still, we doubt her. This will become one of the most difficult aspects of this journey to think about. Alex struggles—afraid and in pain—and nobody believes her. Not even her parents. Alex expresses this in some diary entries.

May 16, 2008

Dear Diary,

My mom says that I am a baby and she looks stupider than I do!!!!!

—Alex

As if it isn't bad enough that she feels I don't support her, she feels the same way about Marc.

May 17, 2008

Dear Diary,

It's not only mom it is dad too uggg both my parents are stupid!!!!!!

—Alex

Something strange seems to happen with Alex's leg: the pain changes. Her leg even begins to look different. When she tries to straighten it, her knee seems to twist inward. Her right knee feels colder than the other. It looks darker, almost purple, and even has more hair on it than her left knee. Alex complains of burning pain. She is sensitive to touch and temperature. She stops wearing pants or letting anything, or anyone, touch her knee. Even a slight amount of wind on her knee sends her into fits of pain.

July 9, 2008

Dear Diary,

I am afraid there is really something wrong with my leg. I am going to see a doctor tomorrow morning.

—Alex

As most parents tend to do, whether they should or not, Marc and I turn to the Internet for information. We look up everything we can. We come across something referred to as both RSD and CRPS. RSD stands for reflex sympathetic dystrophy and CRPS stands for complex regional pain syndrome. They refer to the same condition. Alex's new pain symptoms seem to fit closely with RSD/CRPS. The onset of her illness doesn't make sense but we are grasping at straws.

3

A Diagnosis

It is July 10, 2008, and today we have an appointment with a doctor in Tampa, Florida, who specializes in diagnosing and treating RSD. He speaks kindly to Alex and seems to truly listen to her.

"Tell me about your pain."

Alex is afraid to respond at first; she doesn't trust doctors anymore. "My leg feels sort of burny. It is hot and cold at the same time. I can't stand to have anything touch it. My back feels bad too."

"I'd like to measure the temperatures of both your legs to compare them. Do you mind if I take a close look at them?" After a fairly long examination, the doctor says that Alex has RSD. He speaks to Marc and me about what this means while Alex waits in the reception area.

Alex begins speaking with the receptionist, who is in a wheelchair. Alex is drawn to her. For me, seeing someone with a condition similar to Alex's horrifies me. Alex connects with the woman immediately. Here is someone like her, someone who can understand her. The two of them talk together for quite some time even though Alex is just a child. She has always been able to communicate with adults but this connection seems far

deeper than that. Alex has been forced to grow up over the past
six months. She had been a carefree child and now she is an old
soul in pain. The contrast in her fourth-grade journal entries
over six months of time, from before she got sick to a few months
later, are startling. As part of a class assignment she is required
to write journal entries to family members.

November 1, 2007

Dear Dad,

    I got a new job in class. I have been learning about frac-
tions! I am doing awesome. I have been reading my 5th
Sunshine State book. Plus I am half way done with it. I have
been reading some research I found on the Internet about
tethering dogs and cats. I am highlighting the important
things that I read. I am also training Buttons to be in Pet
Star so I am going to try it next year. I always knew that he
was special!

    I am glad they banned football from recess. I am assistant
go-fer! That is my new job. It turns out that I did not lose my
library book. They returned it! That was all about my week.

—Love, Alex D.

    Her journal entry in November is filled with the types of
things that eleven-year-old children should focus on. Schoolwork,
pets, and plans. There is a great contrast between the entry above
and her journal entry in May. It is all about pain.

Friday, May 23, 2008

Dear Mom,

    I wish my hurting would stop and I know that it is all up
to me but I really wish it wasn't. I like how my PT wanted to

go paint pottery with me. That made my day!!! Although she does hurt me I would rather work with her than anyone else. I wish I could tell her how much I appreciate her. I sort of wish that I could have more fun! I was not here [in school] a lot this week so I don't really know what is going on. I don't know why but I am feeling really, really overwhelmed! I am kind of sad. I miss the days when I ran, jumped, and played, but the most important lesson that I learned is that I am lucky no matter how unlucky you feel because it could be worse.

—Alex

After the RSD doctor examines Alex, he speaks with Marc and me. He tells us there is a measurable difference in temperature between Alex's right leg and her left leg. Her right leg differs physically from her left—a result of RSD. We have a diagnosis. Alex has RSD in her right knee and lower back.

But most RSD is caused from an injury, not an illness. The doctor said that it is useless to try to determine how and why Alex has RSD. Now we just need to focus on helping her with the RSD pain. We want more answers. Alex's symptoms began with an illness. She did not have this strange nerve pain to start. Well, maybe in her lower back. Could it have spread? Could she have had an injury as well? Could we have injured her while trying to straighten her leg during therapy or at home? Had we done this by pushing Alex too hard, by forcing her to try to straighten a leg that wasn't capable of straightening? This is a clear possibility. And so we are still missing something; why wouldn't her leg straighten prior to the pain? So many unanswered questions. In trying to "fix" Alex, we may have made her so much worse. The RSD begins to take center stage. The pain is almost impossible for Alex to bear. Maybe RSD was the culprit all along. Regardless, our efforts turn to helping resolve this pain so Alex can have her life back.

The treatments this doctor suggests seem dramatic and permanent. He speaks of nerve blocks, strong medications, and even cutting nerves in her spinal cord—serious suggestions from a doctor in a little office whom we had never even heard of before our Internet search. This doctor writes a prescription for a wheelchair. He says Alex will likely need it soon. He is right. Shortly after our visit, Alex begins using a wheelchair for long distances. At this point we just accept the change as a natural progression of her illness. It is almost a relief to use the wheelchair to have a way to get Alex around rather than having her hop everywhere. Are we giving in? We question ourselves about this often but we don't stop searching for help.

Our search results in learning about a pain clinic specifically for children with diagnoses of RSD. This impressive clinic is part of a highly respected hospital in New England. This is certainly not a little office with an unknown doctor. What a find!

Going North

I want to contact the director of the clinic—a professor at a major medical school cited all over the Web as an expert in RSD. He is. He is even on the board of directors for the association formed by the doctor in Tampa. I look up his email through the medical school's website and send him an email briefly describing Alex's condition and asking for information about the clinic. As it turns out, I am heading to a town near this hospital tomorrow on a business trip to work on a committee with other mathematics educators from around the country. Maybe I can check out the clinic. Maybe I can even meet with the director. It can't hurt to ask. I find that physicians intimidate people and I don't understand it. I don't feel that same sort of intimidation.

I email him on a Saturday and he sends me a response within the hour! This must be a good omen. I run outside where Marc is setting up a four-foot-high aboveground pool we just purchased at a department store to see if we can use it to help Alex walk. We hope the water will provide the buoyancy so Alex will not need to withstand her own weight but can at least accomplish the mechanics of walking. Marc constantly brainstorms ways to help Alex. We try everything. I come running outside as if we've won the lottery. It feels better than the lottery. We have just found a top-notch clinic that will heal Alex and the director emailed me back on a Saturday! Marc and I feel a surge of hope that we haven't experienced in many months. When we tell Alex, her response is much more guarded. She has been hurt so much by this point that she doesn't get her hopes up like Marc and I do. Maybe her hope has run out. Maybe she feels too much pain to feel other emotions. She still does what we ask. When the pool is finally full, she tries to walk in it. It doesn't work but not because she doesn't try. Marc and I feel disappointed but Alex takes disappointment in stride. I feel sure that this clinic can turn her around and bring back our Alex.

Through emailing with the director I arrange a time to talk on the phone with someone at the clinic on Monday. I don't tell the director I will actually be in the area at the time of our scheduled call. However, I pack all of Alex's medical files in my luggage.

The phone conversation is amazing. This clinic seems like the perfect fit. There are only two issues: a months-long waiting list (the clinic can only serve four children at a time) and a huge price tag. It is unlikely our insurance company will cover it. Marc and I decide to move ahead and worry about finances later. How can we put a price on Alex's wellness?

I persist in saying we will pay cash to cover the cost while we work for insurance coverage. I send messages to relatives putting them on alert that we might need financial help and fast. I tell the clinic I am actually in the area and that we can get to the office with almost no notice. I neglect to tell them that when I say I am in the area I am being quite literal. I let them assume that Alex is with me. I don't want them to perceive any barriers. We just have to get into that clinic. They say that they might have a cancellation due to lack of insurance coverage. If I can get my daughter's files to their office today, Alex might be able to be considered for next week. I say that won't be a problem and hang up. I have no car; I have no idea how to get in to the city where the hospital is located—how am I going to pull this off?

I attend my meeting with seven colleagues from around the country. I share my dilemma with them and they immediately begin figuring out a plan to get me into the city. Ed, a colleague, offers to go with me. We catch a train into the city and a bus from the train station to the doctor's office. We make it just in time to drop off the files. Then we are told that Alex will need to be here for a pre-intake appointment tomorrow. We say no problem and I make arrangements on my cell phone the entire trip back out of the city. Ed calls airlines while I call home. My first call is to my mom.

"Mom, the New England doctor will see Alex tomorrow!"

"Fantastic! What do you need me to do?"

"I need you to drive to the science camp and pick up Alex, take her home and pack her bag, then drive straight to the airport in Orlando. You have to leave right away or you won't make it. I'll meet you at the airport—Ed will drive me. You and Alex will stay with me in my hotel room tonight. We will take the train into the city in the morning. Can you handle Alex and her wheelchair on your own? Flying won't be easy. I think the pressure will hurt her leg even more."

"We'll be fine. I need to go now. I just finished working out and I have to go home and pack before I get Alex. How long will we be there?"

"Just one night. Mom, you have to hurry."

My mom takes everything in stride. She and my dad help us out tremendously. Traveling with Alex is difficult; even getting Alex's wheelchair into my mom's small car is an ordeal. My mom either does it herself or feels comfortable enough to ask strangers to help her. She is so open and friendly that anyone will help her with anything. She has this twinkle in her eye that is unstoppable.

However, this trip puts my mom to the test. They arrive quite late. Ed and I are waiting at the airport as we see Alex and my mom come out of the elevator at baggage claim. They look exhausted and we rush to help them. The flight was as difficult as I anticipated. Alex is in extreme pain but they are here. This is really going to work! Alex and I share the bed and Mom is on the foldout couch, and we fall asleep as soon as our heads hit the pillows. The three of us make the same trek into the city in the morning although it feels quite different taking the train and bus with someone in a wheelchair. Viewing the world through the lens of someone who is physically disabled is a majorly eye-opening experience for me.

It is difficult to get on the train. I try to position Alex's wheelchair so it is out of the traffic pattern on the train. There is a space for wheelchairs but people stand in the area, making it difficult to fit Alex. The train is full. There is no good place for me to stay near Alex and that feels uncomfortable. I want to be by her side.

Getting from the train to the bus is also difficult. We can't find the elevator to get out of the train station—just the escalator but that won't help. We finally find the elevator but then we have to let the bus driver know that he needs to lower the lift so Alex can get on the bus. People are trying to get to work and they don't seem too happy that we are slowing down their commute. I wonder how Alex feels about this. She looks stoic. I wonder how people who deal with commuting in a wheelchair feel every day. I hope that won't be Alex.

We are able to visit the doctors' offices but not the clinic; there is just not enough time. Alex sees an anesthesiologist (the director), a rheumatologist, and a psychologist. Unfortunately, the actual clinic is not in the city but in a neighboring town. There is no way to make it to both locations in the time we have. Still, the visit is very informative and it seems as though the clinic will be an excellent fit for Alex. We are thrilled. It is July 15. They say that there might be an opening at the clinic but Alex will need to be there on July 21 and be prepared to stay for about three weeks. The clinic is an outpatient clinic. The children spend Monday through Friday from eight a.m. to five p.m. in the clinic but do not spend the night, so we will need to find a place to stay and we will need a car to get to and from the clinic. Things are moving so fast, but at least they are moving in the right direction.

My mother and Alex fly home in the evening. I am able to get in to visit the clinic two days later. While there, they tell me there is, in fact, an opening but we will need to pay cash to start at the clinic. The fee is pretty large but we're in! Marc writes a check for $12,000 to cover the first week of therapy. How are we going to come up with $24,000 more for the remaining two weeks? It is a huge shock to write a check like that but we are actually happy to do it. Alex is going to get better. I fly back home right away and begin packing for Alex's trip. Marc plans to drive Alex from Florida all the way up to New England the upcoming weekend. This will allow us to bring whatever we want and it will also provide us with a car while avoiding the expense of a rental for this extended period. The trip is 1,400 miles long. I can't drive with them because I have to give a talk in St. Augustine, Florida, on Monday and it is too late to cancel it. Besides, we really need the money I will make from giving the talk. We are about to go into some major debt.

I arrange to leave directly from my talk to drive to the airport in Orlando and fly to Marc and Alex. I feel so guilty about not making the drive with Alex. I also feel a bit panicked about losing control of even the slightest part of her care. This is a feeling I will continue to experience throughout the entire journey. At one time I complain that I have to handle everything, while simultaneously I complain about others doing things differently from how I might do them. I don't know how Marc can stand me at times. On my part, it is a tough balance. I need to figure out a way to keep my career moving forward while living in a state of uncertainty and concern about Alex. I do think my career plays a large part in keeping me sane. I work mostly with elementary and middle school mathematics teachers, sometimes principals and supervisors. I help them to understand mathematics for teaching. That might sound strange because don't we all feel like we know how to multiply? However, to teach multiplication well, it isn't enough to just know how to multiply, we need to be able to justify why each of the steps in multiplication makes sense. As teachers, we need to make sense of ways students might multiply differently from how we learned and we need to have the number sense to recognize students' errors and correct them on the spot. The expert teacher can anticipate the errors students will make before they even make them. In these ways, knowing mathematics for teaching is quite different from simply knowing mathematics. I just love helping teachers make sense of the mathematics they teach. Often I have the privilege of teaching teachers' students while the teachers watch; this is called model teaching. Teachers find it helpful to get a firsthand account of how to put this knowledge of mathematics for teaching to work for students. I find it helpful to stay current in my practice of teaching children rather than teaching solely adults. I can lose myself in my work for short periods of time, especially when giving presentations. They take all my concentration. It provides some necessary relief. I find ways to avoid too much guilt by saying we need the money from my work to support Alex and we certainly need the insurance. This time, though, as it would be the case many times in the not-too-distant future, it is very difficult to let go and let someone else take care of Alex, even though I will arrive to take back control in just two days.

I will arrive Monday evening. We arrange for Marc to fly home on Tuesday evening to be with Jessica and return to work. My parents come to stay with Jessica as they have on so many occasions throughout this ordeal.

The long drive goes well for Marc and Alex. While they drive, my mother calls every hotel in the area surrounding the clinic. She explains our situation and gets the best rate possible. She reserves a suite at an extended stay hotel, meaning it has a small kitchen. We are in good shape. Now all that is left is for the clinic to fix Alex.

Marc

I don't think I appreciate enough how Marc supports our journey. I get so focused on the search to find help for Alex, ways to provide Jessica some sense of normalcy, and how I am going to balance my girls' needs with my work responsibilities that I don't stop to think that Marc is doing the same thing. Marc lets me take the lead but he does so much as well, just not in the spotlight.

Marc is an engineer, a problem solver. He doesn't always think that he is a great parent but he is. He loves his family; we are all he seems to need. Other than at work, he does not spend time with people outside of our family and he is fulfilled. Since Alex got sick, he spends hours and hours researching illnesses with symptoms related to hers. Because I am a professor, we have access to the university library. He searches through medical research journals. If he cannot access them through my library, he searches using engineering search engines. As a contractor for NASA, he works at the Kennedy Space Center. Between the university library and the library at the Kennedy Space Center, he has plenty to read. When he finds information he thinks might be useful, he highlights it and asks me to read it so we can discuss it. We are a team.

He doesn't think he is a good enough parent because he feels he loses his patience too quickly—and sometimes he does. But our situation is not just difficult but desperate. I don't have to worry about leaving Jessica when I accompany Alex at the clinic. I know Marc will be fine with her. They will surely eat more spaghetti than usual but Jessica will have help with her homework, she will have conversation over dinner, her laundry will be clean, and she will be safe. She will have hugs when she needs them and a lunch to bring to school. Marc always does fine with the girls when I travel. They have fun together. They almost always go out for pizza at least once while I am away—something we rarely do when I am home. They argue at times but I think that is normal.

Marc grew up in Miami. He is handsome, almost six feet tall, thin, and naturally muscular with distinguished early gray hair. He loves warm weather, sunny beaches, and sailing. He is happiest when sailing. We spend great weekends on our sailboat. It's not fancy and somewhat old but it offers a true getaway and provides an amazing environment for family time. Before Alex got sick, we spent most weekends on the boat. We would sail or go to the beach during the day and play games or rent movies and watch them in the evening. After Alex got sick, we stopped sailing. We tried to go at first but the wind hurt Alex's leg and she found it almost impossible to maneuver on the boat. Without a place to de-stress, Marc's blood pressure climbs. Eventually he has to start taking blood pressure medication. Though his hair started turning gray in high school, I know for a fact he is getting much grayer during Alex's illness.

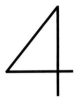

The Pain Clinic

Beginning at the clinic is a bit of a rude awakening. We drive to the back of the hospital, park, enter onto a long hallway that is sort of a ramp, turn the corner at the bottom, and there is the clinic. It has a small waiting area and a glass door marking the clinic entrance. There are window stickers of sea animals on the glass. It looks inviting and friendly. That is clearly a façade. You can't just walk into the clinic—you have to be let in—and parents aren't allowed. The clinic coordinator meets the kids at the door promptly at eight a.m. and says good-bye to the small collection of parents with a stern look and what I guess is an Irish accent. She is abrupt with us; the way she looks at us makes me feel almost guilty, like it is our fault that our children are in pain and disabled. Before I leave, I witness the wheelchair being taken from Alex. She is told she no longer needs it—using a wheelchair will not be tolerated—but Alex can't walk. I start to protest but I am given a look so severe I stop midsentence. For a moment I want to take Alex away from the coordinator and carry her to the car; leaving her here is a mistake! Before I can act the door closes and Alex is gone. I just stand there. Now what?

The first day passes so slowly. I go back to the hotel and pace. I try to do some work I brought but it is no use. I can't wait to get Alex at five o'clock. I am waiting at the door with the sea stickers, peering through the glass trying to catch a glimpse of Alex ten minutes before five.

"How was it?"

"Awful. I hate it. I want to go home. How am I supposed to get to the car?"

"I don't know." Alex begins to hop. It takes fifteen minutes just to get to the car. I feel so bad for her. I want to carry her again but I know that will not be acceptable. This is how things will be. Alex hops everywhere and she is miserable.

One of four children in the program, Alex is by far the youngest. The ages range from ten to seventeen years old. Children graduate out of the program after making a reasonable level of progress and children on the waiting list take their place. While Alex is there, an eight-year-old girl enters the clinic as well. These children had been figure skaters, soccer players, dancers, football players, and skiers, and then an injury, often a mild one, stops them in their tracks. They are no longer able to participate in their sports or even attend school due to the incapacitating pain this disorder causes. The affected limb often becomes twisted or otherwise distorted. How could I have never heard of this disorder before? How are these kids going to get their lives back? This clinic is designed to help them and everyone in it means business.

Alex has physical therapy, occupational therapy, group therapy, and individual psychological therapy every day. The team works her hard. Sometimes it seems like torture. In order to help her to get used to the nerve pain in her leg, the occupational therapist rubs different substances on her leg—from lotion to marbles to sand. The physical therapists try to get her to straighten her leg and put weight on it. The psychologist works on helping Alex to ignore the pain so it won't rule her life. Alex keeps a journal the entire visit. The entries she makes speak volumes.

Wednesday, July 23, 2008

Dear Diary,

Today was my third day of torture at the clinic and let me tell you it is not easy. See I have RSD and it is very hard! I am in a nine hour a day physical therapy five days a week and let me tell you they don't take no as an answer!!! You might feel tired now but there we dream of getting a one minute break. It is really hard to get out of a wheelchair and into a walker. I work with three other girls and I have the farthest to go to get better it feels like. Believe in your self it helps a lot!

—Alex

Alex comes home just miserable every day. Home is actually the hotel but it begins to feel like our home. We put photos of our family, friends, and pets all over the walls to help us feel less homesick. I try to establish routines to help Alex feel more comfortable in this new place. However, Alex becomes more and more withdrawn. She has her own room and she wants to escape to it frequently. She just isn't improving. She doesn't feel good about herself.

Tuesday, July 29, 2008

Dear Diary,

People think that I can do things that I cannot. I am supposed to get better quickly but I am not. I am mad, sad, angry, and scared.

—Bye, Alex

The clinic team says she needs to be more motivated. I must admit I find myself agreeing with them. They are the experts. If they say she isn't working hard enough, then it must be true. They send her home with therapy assignments to complete each day. This is after a grueling nine-hour day at the clinic. We get back to the hotel and Alex hops through the lobby to the elevator and then to our rooms. I go back downstairs to see what food the hotel puts out for social hour and try to make a meal out of it for us, supplementing with whatever groceries we have. Then we start on the list of homework tasks. We do some of them in our rooms and others in the hotel hallway, depending on what is required. I'm sure the hotel staff and guests find us curious. Alex does some strange homework. She might have to try to walk like a crab on her hands and feet—not my favorite, as it is all I can do to push the idea that she is dragging herself along a disgusting hotel hallway out of my mind. She might have to stand on both feet to draw a picture. This sounds strange until you realize that she no longer lets her right foot touch the ground unless pushed to do so. She often has to massage lotion into her right knee. You would think this one would be easy but just touching her knee is often more than Alex can handle. She gave up on sleeping with even a sheet on her leg months ago.

I attack the list with a vengeance. Alex just *has to* begin improving. It seems to me that she is trying at home with me but I don't see improvement there either.

Friday, August 1, 2008

Dear Diary,

It is Friday!!! I got things put in my shoes today. Uggg my leg really hurts!!! I really wish it would stop hurting. I do

not get why I am not making more progress but I will just
have to wait to turn the corner.

—Alex

She picks a theme song to support her; choosing theme songs
will become a trend. Her theme song is "Lean on Me." I don't
think she has anyone to lean on in the clinic. Maybe she leans
on the other children. At times, I suppose she leans on me. We
do find opportunities to laugh but they are mostly during the
weekends when the clinic is closed. We explore the nearby city
and its surrounding areas. One weekend we go whale watching.
I have to carry Alex onto the boat. This is no small feat as she
is nearly my height. I sort of place her over my shoulder; I don't
know how else to do it. A man sees me struggling and carries her
part of the way. I'm both mortified and relieved. She is in too
much pain to really enjoy it but I don't want her to stop living
so we do it anyway. We spend some time with the other families
affected by RSD. These families suffer as well. This pain disorder
can tear you apart. One mom struggles with her husband leaving
her while she is with us at the clinic. It is easy to see how this
can happen. If both parents aren't on the same page regarding
this disorder, I don't know how their marriage can survive it
intact. There is no guidebook for this all-consuming journey.

Another mom decides to relocate her entire family from
Texas to a town near the clinic just to be near doctors who
seem to understand this awful disorder. She leaves a thriving
veterinary practice behind. These women become my support
group. Their children and Alex develop a strong bond. They
have all faced people who think they are malingering for attention. They have faced doctors who have said, "I've never seen

anything like this," as my daughter has heard so many times. Those doctors left the children feeling like freaks or worse: liars. It is helpful for Alex and me to spend time away from the clinic with people who understand our plight. We focus on healing during these weekends. We lean on one another. This isn't the case on weekdays when the clinic is the main focus. I want to find ways to support Alex's efforts to show her I believe in her. We go online and create yellow rubber bracelets that say RESILIENCE STRENGTH DETERMINATION to represent what we feel Alex needs to overcome this thing called RSD that has taken over her life. We order them and Alex sends the bracelets to everyone she knows. She writes the following letter to describe what it is like to have RSD.

Sunday, August 3, 2008

Hi,

I'm writing this letter to tell you about what my life is like with Reflex Sympathetic Dystrophy or RSD. Most people don't know or recognize what RSD is. I think because it's not a disease that can kill you or a disease that can be fixed by a doctor. But it can make your life not worth living. It is hard to live with because it kind of stops the cycle of living and feeling of other things and yourself. But the best thing you can do is believe you will get better, because believing makes all the difference.

I am in a pain center. I work harder than I imagined every day. It is the most painful thing I could ever imagine. It feels like a hot/cold sensation that is inside you that never stops. It throbs and burns all the time. I have it in my knee but other kids at the center have it in their feet, arms, and shoulders. When I got here I was in a wheelchair. Now I use a walker but I cannot use my leg very well. I am working on it. It is very painful and it feels like my leg is stuck. I can't move it and I can't seem to feel my muscles to signal them to move. I have to retrain my brain to feel the muscles and know how to manipulate them. I do that by doing things over and over again. I have two physical therapists push my leg down while I stand on a scale to push down 50 pounds. No matter how much I scream and cry, I have to keep going.

You can help me by spreading the news about RSD. I am sending you a bracelet that says Resilience Strength Determination. It is what I need to get over RSD. People who don't know about RSD think people like me aren't telling the truth when we talk about our pain. That is really hard. You can help by learning more about it and sharing what you know.

—Alex

I hadn't heard of RSD before Alex's illness. How many other people suffer with RSD and never find out what it is? How many people never get help? We are able to rely on family to help us to bring Alex to a well-respected clinic. While it is a financial stretch, we are able to pay for a hotel room for all the time we are here. My husband and often my parents are able to stay home with Jessica, and my job allows me to work remotely for extended periods of time. My parents stay with Jessica quite a bit during Alex's illness. When I need to leave for work, my mother flies to Alex to take my place. That sort of family support is unusual. My mom is able to step right in and take over almost seamlessly. I know how lucky we are to have such support.

Grandma

It isn't until my mom has been with Alex at the clinic for a few days while I am traveling for work do I begin to speak to the other moms of the kids at the clinic. Mom paves the way for me by striking up conversations and getting to know them first. My mother asks them to go for coffee one morning after bringing Alex to the clinic; I just wouldn't have thought to do that. I may never have developed these relationships that become so important without my mom's help. My mother not only sees the cup as half full, but overflowing. She can befriend anyone.

My mother is amazing. There is no other way to say it. She is seventy years old, although you would never know it by looking at her—or by trying to keep up with her for that matter. She is proud of her age because she doesn't feel it or look it. She still works out several times per week. Her favorites are Zumba, Pilates, and yoga. She also likes to figure skate. She was a dancer as a child and she maintains the presence of someone who has performed. She is only five foot two but her personality is much bigger than that.

Alex and Jessica like to do crafts. We need my mother for that department as well as I am not crafty. I can't even wrap a birthday present. Marc and I keep a large plastic box of gift bags under our bed at home—the girls know that presents from us are put in gift bags—the same gift bags over and over again with the same crumpled tissue paper from last year, no bows, no frilly ribbons. I cook the same things over and over again too. Grocery lists are easy; they are exactly the same from one week to the next: grilled chicken with broccoli, grilled chicken with asparagus, fish with string beans, repeat. I don't sew; when I was in graduate school, too far away from my mom, there were times that I used a stapler to hem my pants. I don't even like to shop. Every Valentine's Day I take the same two stuffed animals with hearts on them that I've given the girls every Valentine's Day since they were little and put them someplace in the house for the girls to come upon. I might put them in their beds at night, on their bathroom counter, at their places at the table. The girls pretend they are excited and surprised and they sleep with them that evening, then I pack them away for the next year. I do all this to avoid shopping for something new each year. I think Jessica only recently realized I was using the same animals over year after year and that was just because Alex told her.

My mom likes to shop. She does all these sorts of things with my daughters. We count on her for it. She can make anything. The girls love everything she cooks. She always has a knitting bag with her; she knits the most beautiful sweaters. She was teaching Alex to knit around the time Alex got sick.

My mom was an elementary school teacher for years and years. She has a way with children that can't be beat. My girls adore her. Whenever I have to travel from the clinic my mom flies in the night before and effortlessly steps into my shoes. This allows life to go on in some capacity that would not be possible otherwise. I do my best to maintain my career while supporting Alex. I need it for the money, the insurance, and probably most important, my sanity. Jessica needs people to focus on her when I cannot. My mom knows all of these things and does what needs to be done. She steps into my shoes at home as well, keeping Jessica's life as stable as possible given the circumstances.

HOT POTATO (BY JESSICA DIXON)

Mom was on a work trip then the next thing you know Alex is picked up by Grandma to go fly to a hospital then to my shock they are back the next day. Right after that Alex is stolen from me again. I just watch Alex and Dad pack the car feeling left out. I wish I could go too but what help would me going be? Alex is always kind of sad nowadays. It is like she gave up on life. Yet, my brave older sister still puts on a mask to hide the pain around me. She pretends it is all good and sits down to play dolls with me. Dolls were almost all we played once her illness started since she could no longer play outside. Still I can see through it. Most of all I can see it in her eyes. Her eyes are always sad now. They are missing that familiar twinkle of heart and happiness. The muffled sobbing in her room at night lets me know as well. What scared me really bad that showed how much pain she was in at the time is when I accidentally touched her bad leg. She started crying like the time she broke her elbow but the way she cried it sounded like she was in worse pain than that.

Mom, Alex, and Dad left me with Grandma and Grandpa. Dad and Grandma go back and forth a lot. I wonder if the clinic is working. Well of course it would work. It is an RSD clinic after all. To me at least, it almost seems like it is made for my big sister. My grandparents said I might get to visit Alex and Mom soon. I hope so and I hope this is the longest I will be without them. Grandma said that we are going to visit my Aunt Marni in Maryland. I miss my cousin Taylor but I would much rather see Alex. I feel like I am going to go on a vacation. They pretend it is one, but in my heart I know the truth. They don't know what to do with me. I almost feel like a hot potato. I feel like something that they can't keep for long, or don't want to keep for long. For me a vacation is a break not a distraction from the truth. It is something I rather not do alone but with my family. This is not a vacation but something to keep me from the drama and pain. That causes me to feel pained and abandoned. I wish they knew it doesn't help. I wish I could be with them. What they don't understand is that knowing the cold hard truth is better than being in the dark. They will heal Alex without me being a part of it or even being there. That's enough to ruin someone's "vacation" right?

When I get to Maryland I have a lot of fun. I go ice skating, and to the beach! I go to see Aunt Marni's house for the first time since I was a baby! Taylor is so lucky! She has a bird named Perry, a bunch of fish, a basement filled with arcade games, and a beach house. I know I am luckier; Taylor doesn't have a sister and I have the best one of all.

Alex will even get to run and play with me after the clinic. Alex and me used to invite people from the neighborhood and play freeze tag. When she comes home we will push each other on the swing and jump off when Mom's not looking. Maybe we will even invite the boy we both have a MAJOR crush on to play with us. Just like the old times. I remember like it was yesterday when Alex was going to the doctors because of her back pain. I also remember in painful clarity when I came inside from playing with my neighbor on the swing set. When I came in my dad was waiting there with an arm to cry on and the news that Alex was in the hospital. It was only the start of bad news. One of the worst memories I have is visiting my happy, beautiful Alex at the hospital but there she wasn't happy and she was still beautiful on the outside but missing that inner glow. She was a shadow of her former self. She was an empty shell. Alex was missing that spark of life. Now she is surviving without living and wishing she wasn't surviving. That will all change when she is done with the clinic.

I leave Aunt Marni's to go visit Alex. By now I am sick of the driving. It was a seventeen-hour drive to Maryland and the next thing you know I am off to somewhere else. I get so carsick I have to bring a pail to throw up in. It is a cute purple-colored sand bucket that smells like puke. No matter how many times we wash it, that smell never comes out. It is supposed to keep me from throwing up all over the car but there have been some mishaps. Mom's car often smells like the bucket. It is fondly referred to as the "puke bucket." I had to use that bucket four times on my drive up and after this trip I will have to drive back home. I still want to see Alex and see how she improved. I wonder if she is out of her wheelchair.

When I get there I meet Zombie Alex. Her spark has done more than died. The spark froze. She is tired and skinny. If you saw her without knowing her she would look dreadfully ill. In a way she is dreadfully ill. She hops rather than walks to get around and looks like she really needs a wheelchair. That fire of hope inside of me is devoured by disappointment. All that is left is a small flicker. The undoubted idea of a full recovery becomes much more doubted. If anything, Alex looks worse. But maybe it will work, I tell myself. I continue to lie to spare my heart.

When I get to the hotel, I really like it. It is more like home than our own house at the moment. People say home is where the heart is. That is true. My heart lies with my family so where my family is, my home is. The suite is cozy and themed in a deep blue color. Pictures of our family are pinned to the walls. This place has more pictures of Alex and me on the walls than our house. I guess they miss me as much as I miss them. It is nice to know they think about me, but it doesn't help much when I want them to be with me. I like the view and it serves as a minihouse. It doesn't feel like a hotel room.

There is more of a connection to this cluster of rooms than an average hotel room. I love sharing a room with Alex. It is the first time Alex and I share a room since the townhouse we rented before we moved to our house. Even though she is an empty shell, I still love that shell. Even though it isn't truly Alex, it is more of her than I had for a while and I cherish it. I also really miss Mom and Dad. For the rest of that day, I am flipping over from disappointment to joy.

I am pleased to find a fish in the suite. Mom and Zombie Alex bought a deep blue beta fish to keep them company. It fits in just right, matching the color and feel of the room. Alex leaves to go to the clinic each morning. It sounds like torture, but it is made for my sister to get better so maybe it is Alex just being reluctant. After Mom and Alex get home from the clinic, we go to the pet store. I am going to get a beta fish and I will get a cute tank just like Alex's. The beta fish is a beautiful deep blue with a top fin colored a brilliant red. It stands out among the beta fish with fin disease and incompatible coloring. I just have to have it. So I pick up the beautiful fish's bag with poop-filled water and buy it.

Mom has to run to a department store to buy something. We are in the middle of the store when some of the poop water gets on me. Not only do I puke when I get carsick, I puke when things are gross. I find that gross and puke in the middle of the store. I just sit there watching the frantic rush of my mother trying to clean up my mess with paper towels. If I didn't still have poop water on me, I would find it funny. We leave the bag with the fish at the hotel and we go out to dinner. I don't like most of the meals on the menu. My mom thinks I will like Caesar salad so she orders it for me. Now my beautiful fish is still without a name. I really like this Caesar salad. Our waitress comes to our table to see if we need anything and I tell her what my fish's name is. I named it Caesar. The young waitress eager to listen to the cute eight-year-old (who looks more like five) asks if I named it after the Roman leader. Jokes on her, I named it after my new favorite salad.

I have to leave my family again. I can only spend a week with them. In this one week, I am able to get a fish and visit the aquarium. I will really miss my family. Now I am leaving in the car. I am reacquainting with the "puke bucket." I might be away from my family now, but I will be with them when my fully recovered sister comes back. Well, at least I tell myself that.

··

A Change in Focus

Eventually, insurance agrees to cover the clinic. That is a huge relief. However, in order to maintain coverage, the clinic has to show that Alex is improving. They find ways to demonstrate she is improving on assessments they give her. I meet with the team once per week to review the results and talk about goals. We sit around a conference table in a small room and each doctor or therapist gives his or her report. I feel like what they say is fake. I feel like my questions, such as, "How specifically is she improving because I just don't see it?" are not appreciated. Nor do I think they are answered honestly. I do not miss the sideways glances to one another or the therapists squirming slightly in their seats as they answer me, making very little eye contact with me as they do. They say things like, "This week she was able to tolerate fifty pounds of weight on her right leg for ten seconds as opposed to just five seconds last week." This just doesn't seem like reasonable progress to me. She could do that when we arrived. I actually think she is getting worse. I don't see the improvements the team is claiming. I don't let these thoughts go and continue to question them. They keep saying that, while she is not improving at a very good rate, she is improving. They say that we just have to work on her attitude and motivation. Eventually, the psychological support takes center stage.

Tuesday, August 5, 2008

Dear Diary,

Uggg it is sooo hard to say what you feel. Because it is sooo hard to express the pain and misery that I am going through . . . .

—Alex

It seems that efforts turn to trying to uncover a reason for her to want to maintain her current condition. What happened in her past that would make her want to stay sick? I don't think anything happened. But once again, they are the experts . . . .

Monday, August 11, 2008

Dear Diary,

I am beginning to feel alone and I know that my mom is the best but I just sometimes cannot keep up with time. I am in soooooooooooooooo much PAIN!!! I wish I could take my mind off it better. I tried to put my foot down today but it is soooo hard ugg but I have to keep trying if I want to get better . . . .

—Alex

Alex doesn't think anything happened to make her want to be like this either but she decides to take the psychologists for a ride. If they think she is a psychological mess, then she will give them something to talk about. She is a very smart girl. She leads them on a wild goose chase into her past. She has them exploring all sorts of ridiculous topics. I am horrified by her change in behavior but I can't do anything about it. I see that she is acting more and more childish with the therapists at the clinic in ways she does not behave with me. I am frustrated with her and I get angry with her in front of the therapists. I can see that they are watching me to see how I treat Alex. I can't seem to get them to see that they are creating this ridiculous situation.

Tuesday, August 19, 2008

Dear Diary,

I am doing a bunch of things to help me get better like standing on my leg for 5 seconds even though it has been 5 weeks I cannot give up! It is hard because the psychologist keeps saying that there is a mental block that is keeping me from getting better. I just cannot find out what it is. My back is feeling like RSD too and my left leg is swelling because all I am doing is hopping on one leg. Ugg.

—Alex

It is a difficult situation. I know the therapists are wasting precious time looking for whatever they mean by her mental block. We are spending a fortune staying here and we are keeping our family apart. I feel that Alex is trying and I also feel that Alex isn't improving. On top of all of that, I am afraid to leave. We have nowhere else to go. I'm not the only one with these feelings.

Tuesday, August 26, 2008

Dear Diary,

I have been having panic attacks a lot tonight and I am worried about tomorrow and I do want to go home but I want to be better when I go home and I am not making progress so I have to go to a conference. Me and my family are hoping I do not get sent home or I will probably not get better. *Help! Help! Help!*

—Alex

We spend nine weeks in the clinic. When we arrived, Alex couldn't walk. When we leave, she still can't walk well. She develops a very lopsided gait that allows her to walk by putting almost no weight on her right leg. She gets around but not well. I don't think the clinic knows what else to do with her.

Tuesday, September 16, 2008

Dear Diary,

It is my 9th week at the [clinic] and I am leaving in 3 days. I don't think they could keep me any longer and I am not walking yet. They said that if I walk by Friday I get a graduation. If I do not I will just go home. I am trying my hardest . . . .

—Alex

They have a graduation and send her home. They didn't fix her as we had hoped. Alex feels like a failure and I feel so let down. Even though insurance covers the cost of the clinic, our family has lived apart for nine weeks. We spent thousands and thousands of dollars on the hotel and travel. We put our hope, energy, and finances into this plan and we don't feel as though it is a success.

When we first learned about the clinic, there had been talk of follow-up visits. We are not contacted. I hear of other children being contacted and invited for return visits. I feel angry and jealous—what's so wrong with Alex and me that they would give up on us? I am really surprised by the way we are just dropped but then I come to feel less surprised. They are probably relieved to have us leave.

5

Moving On but Not for Long

Alex returns to a school year that is already a month underway. She is in the fifth grade. She has no problem making up the work she missed due to her academic giftedness. After our experience in the clinic, we decide to focus on living as opposed to physical therapy. We work with a psychologist, although we are not sure it is much help. We do not put Alex in physical therapy. She attends school and takes piano lessons. I wouldn't say she is happy and she is certainly still in pain. I'm not sure this way of life can go on indefinitely but we are not given the opportunity to find out.

Alex is still unable to straighten her leg completely or to walk with a normal gait. Her right heel doesn't touch the ground at all when she walks. However, she still wants to fit in. A few months ago she decided that at the one-year mark from the onset of her illness she would be all better. She was sure of it. Well, it is coming up on a year and Alex isn't all better. It is January 2009 and her classmates are jumping rope during physical education class. Alex decides to join them. Because her leg won't straighten, she jumps rope on one leg. She falls and breaks her right heel and the growth plate to her right ankle. They aren't bad breaks.

She is given a soft cast. The breaks just don't seem to heal. Her foot becomes more and more pointed and her heel is farther and farther off the ground. We bring her to her orthopedist and he suggests she return to physical therapy to try to get her to stretch her Achilles tendon. We are back to physical therapy three times per week. However, it is different this time.

Alex's ankle seems to be stuck. Her leg is still strange. When she tries to straighten it, her kneecap turns in so that it faces her other leg. It turns in what seems like an impossible way. Her kneecap points inward and her foot points outward. It is almost like the upper and lower parts of her leg are not connected. Her ankle won't do anything. Her foot is just pointed, almost like a ballerina. Her physical therapist, a very strong man, tries to stretch her ankle with all his might. Alex can carry on a conversation while her PT is breaking into a sweat pulling her foot so hard. It doesn't hurt. It is just stuck. Not only is her foot stuck in a pointed position, her entire right leg seems to be getting weaker and weaker. The PT positions Alex in a leg press where she is to lie on her back and push a flat medal platform with her legs starting out bent and then straightening. She can push a reasonable weight with her left foot but she can't even move the platform without any weight using her right foot. We can't make sense of this. Why is her leg so weak and why is her foot so ridiculously pointed? We even try a splint that uses springs to stretch her ankle all night while she sleeps. The thought is that if we keep a constant stretch for eight hours her ankle will begin to give. What gives is the brace. It just comes off her ankle.

Once again, we feel frightened with nowhere to turn. Her orthopedic doctors don't know what to do. I email the doctors from the pain clinic in New England. Eventually, we have a phone conversation and plan for Alex to make a trip back up north to see the doctors up there again. It is April 2009—seven months since we were last there—and Alex spends two days visiting doctors at the hospital up north and at the pain clinic. She sees an anesthesiologist, a rheumatologist, an orthopedist, and a physical therapist. They are proud of Alex's progress in dealing with her pain. They are not quite sure what to make of her ankle. The only suggestion we come away with is to think about returning to this hospital for what doctors referred to as an intrathecal baclofen test. Alex is already taking baclofen orally, as it is supposed to help with her pain and tightness. I am not convinced it does much of anything. The doctors think if we introduce the baclofen to her spinal fluid, it will do more to loosen her ankle than what can be taken orally because a much higher dose can be used to target the area that needs it. This is an interesting concept but also frightening. It will need to occur during a stay at the hospital there. We decide to explore other options first.

We contact an orthopedic surgeon in Maryland. Some doctors feel that Alex's foot is stuck in the pointed position because her Achilles tendon has shortened. They say she might need surgery to release it. I email a surgeon in Maryland renowned for these sorts of procedures. He emails me back. We speak on the phone and he feels that a new brace—a custom knee device—he and his physical therapist colleague are working on might help. It is mostly used for people with cerebral palsy. We make plans to fly from the appointments up north to see this doctor and physical therapist in Maryland.

When the orthopedist in New England hears we plan to visit this well-known doctor in Maryland, he defers to the Maryland doctor, saying he really doesn't know how to advise us. He has never seen anything like what he sees with Alex. We feel so tired of hearing that. We hope we won't get the same response in Maryland.

And we don't get quite the same response from Maryland but we do get yet another brace—a hinged plaster cast extending from Alex's toes to her thigh. It is open along the top so Alex can remove it during the day but sleep in it at night. Areas on the cast to wrap large rubber straps provide a gentle stretch throughout the night. This should work better than the brace with springs that slipped off because this brace completely encases her leg from high on her thigh to the tip of her toes. There is no way for it to slip off. We fly home with the cast. Alex wears it for the next month with no change. We are beginning to have quite a collection of retired braces. It looks like we need to head back to the New England hospital.

Thursday, May 7, 2009

Dear Journal,

The clinic doctors emailed back. All I really want to do is get mad. They are talking about doing a lot of scary things like MRIs with needles in my hip, baclofen, and epidurals and pumps with surgery. I might be going up there on May 17, 2009, for 8 days to get admitted into the hospital to run tests on me. Sounds exciting, doesn't it? Meanwhile my hip is popping/dislocating and I am freaking out. My contractures and RSD is really bad too. I am sleeping in a huge Custom Knee Device.

People keep looking at me like I am weird. I have had this problem for a year and a half and I am done with it!

—Alex

P.S. I am not weird I am just different.

The Third Time Up North is NOT the Charm

Friday, May 15, 2009

Dear Journal,

I have 2 more days to go until I go back up north to the hospital. I found out that I am going to get an arthrogram, scary. I am going to be in torture next week.

—*Alex*

Marc and I bring Alex back up north to the hospital. With Alex needing to be put under general anesthesia, I feel afraid to take her by myself. Marc has used up a significant amount of sick and vacation time over the last year and a half. We have to make decisions like this carefully. We also don't like to both go and leave Jessica behind. As usual, my parents stay with her. This is a big deal; Alex will have to be placed under general anesthesia. She will need to have something like an epidural, which makes us nervous. Around the time we are heading back up north to the hospital, Alex's right hip starts to do something strange when she walks. It makes this strange popping sound. You can actually see it; it looks like it repeatedly dislocates and goes back into place with a rapid motion. Alex finds that if she sits down she can get the "popping" to stop. We call it popping because we have no idea what else to call it. It is happening more and more frequently. We feel fairly certain her hip is dislocating. The doctor from the clinic does not think it is dislocating. Months later we will know for certain that it had been.

As we are going up the elevator to our hotel room the night before Alex is going to be admitted into the hospital, Alex stands against the inside of the elevator. Her hip begins to pop and bang against the wall of the elevator. It feels like her hip shakes the entire elevator. The sound reverberates and Alex looks to us with pleading eyes. Marc and I look at each other and know we need to be where we are, about to be admitted to this highly respected hospital to explore the next level of treatment.

The process in the hospital begins with a hip arthrogram, as there is some concern that her hip popping is damaging her hip. It is. Her hip is degenerating, resulting in permanent damage! The orthopedist says that she will end up needing a hip replacement at a young age if the degeneration continues. How can we have ended up in this mess? We don't know how to get her hip to stop popping. We have no idea why it is even popping to begin with but if we don't find a way to keep it from happening, Alex's hip will be destroyed. Our focus turns to hoping the intrathecal baclofen test will work.

Even if the test works, we are going down a road we can hardly fathom. The intrathecal baclofen test is just a one-time dose of baclofen introduced to Alex's spinal fluid. If it results in her ankle relaxing, or returning to a normal position, Alex will need surgery to implant a baclofen pump in her abdomen. Just thinking about it feels like we are in the twilight zone. We are actually hoping she will get one of these contraptions!

The hospital admits Alex and the tests begin—and so does the nightmare. The director of the pain clinic from the previous summer is in charge of Alex's case and this procedure. He notes that when under general anesthesia Alex's ankle returns to a normal position. That means her Achilles tendon is not the culprit. It is something else. He takes a picture of her ankle with his cell phone to show Alex (and Marc and me) proof that her ankle can relax. He comes out to the waiting area to show Marc and me the picture while Alex is still under. He almost looks smug—as if to say "I told you so—she can control this." His attitude should have provided me with a better indication of what is to come.

In addition to giving Alex the baclofen, he makes a cast of Alex's foot while it is relaxed under anesthesia. The cast will be cut off and made into a brace for later use. He leaves the cast on. I guess he hopes the baclofen will relax her ankle and her ankle will be able to stay in a neutral position. The cast will need to be cut off as the baclofen dose wears off. She is also given an epidural to use with the cast so she can tolerate the pain over the next several days.

Things do not go smoothly. First, Alex is not told that she will wake up in a cast nor are we. She wakes surprised and afraid to find a cast on her leg as she comes out of anesthesia. Second, the cast really hurts. Marc and I are with her as she wakes up. So is the doctor. The three of us are standing around her hospital bed in recovery. Nurses are doing their work around us seemingly nonplussed by Alex's reaction. She begins crying and carrying on. She screams for us to get the cast off of her. She says the cast is killing her, that it feels like it is breaking her foot. She even tries to pull the cast off herself, which is, of course, impossible. The doctor doesn't seem to believe her. He tells her she needs to wait it out. He shows her the picture of her foot under general anesthesia. He says that she can relax it to a neutral position and that the picture proves it. I am afraid she is going to knock the cell phone right out of his hand. Alex feels betrayed—is she getting "tricked" again, like the neurologist in Orlando tried to do?

Marc and I don't know whom to believe. Our eyes keep meeting, with each of us looking to the other for a hint of what we should do, how we should respond to Alex. She seems like she is in real pain but the doctor just showed us a picture of her foot in a neutral position. Does she just need to wait it out? Is she really in that much pain or is she just scared? Eventually, the cast is cut off to get bivalves for later use. By the time the cast is cut off, Alex's skin around her ankle is raw. Her foot had been pointing with so much force inside her cast that her skin is damaged. Could she have really done that on purpose? It doesn't seem like it.

Alex spends two weeks in the hospital. Marc has to leave to go back to work a few days after we arrive. The entire experience is horrible. The doctor tries to get Alex's foot to loosen by having her wear the bivalve cast with the epidural each night. The nurses and I basically jam the cast onto Alex's leg the best we can and then strap it on. Alex is in so much pain. This eventually causes skin breakdown from her foot pointing inside the cast. We put skin protection on her foot and ankle where there is breakdown to serve as a second skin and continue this ridiculous practice. It is awful.

Nurses ask, "On a scale of zero to ten, describe your pain. Zero means no pain and a ten is the worst pain you could imagine." Alex responds by saying the pain scale is flawed because it is always changing. Just when she thinks she knows what a ten is, her pain gets worse and she has to revise the scale and change all her numbers.

Absolutely miserable, Alex feels disappointed once again. She meets with a psychologist a few times but doesn't find it helpful. He doesn't know her. This psychologist doesn't consult the psychologist from the pain clinic for any background information on Alex. He only knows Alex on the surface, he only knows what she chooses to show him in her current state. He thinks he knows her, but he doesn't . . . .

We aren't the only family from the pain clinic experiencing difficult times at the hospital. The veterinarian's eight-year-old daughter who had been in the pain clinic with Alex is also admitted while we are here. Strangely, her shoulders are "popping" in and out in the same way Alex's hip pops. We have no idea how to explain it nor do the doctors. She actually went to a different emergency room in the area and they didn't know what to do with her so they sent her to the emergency room at this hospital. This emergency room admits her right away. Her shoulders pop so badly she looks like a fish flopping around. She can't feed herself or care for herself. It is awful. What is going on with these children?

It seems that as the girls' joints pop more and more, the doctors become more and more convinced that they must be doing it on purpose. The other girl's mom and I begin comparing notes. We both keep hearing the term "conversion disorder." Conversion disorder is a condition that affects a person's nervous system and often occurs as a result of a psychological conflict. How can our doctors think that? Haven't we been through this before? Are they calling our daughters, and us, liars? The other mom is solid as she stands her ground. She knows this is real. I find myself in turmoil once again. Why do I keep questioning Alex? I know it's real too. My "mother's instinct" speaks to me clearly. Why do I always question what I know is true?

Both our daughters are getting worse. We are in what we believed to be one of the best hospitals in the country. The other mom relocated her entire family to the area to be closer to this hospital, and they are saying this is all in our daughters' heads. It is unbelievable. And it is about to get worse.

The Meeting

About a week or so into our stay, a very disturbing thing happens. I have been staying in Alex's room with her. It is not a private room. We even have to share the bathroom. We feel lucky because a few days ago our roommate went home and we got permission to change sides of the room. We moved away from the door to the side that has the bathroom. It is so much better to be able to use the bathroom without feeling like intruders on the other patient's space, even if we do have to walk through her space to get in and out of the room. We don't leave often.

The room is so cramped. I stay on a reclining chair next to Alex's bed. We have to place all of our things on the windowsill behind the chair. I just stack it all up, essentially covering the window but there is no place else to put it. When I recline the chair, the floor space is completely covered. I have to climb into the chair over its arm. I don't know how a less agile parent would manage—maybe that is why I don't see too many other parents staying here. I just climb over the arm, wrap myself in a blanket so I won't feel the vinyl of the chair against my skin, and attempt to sleep in a strange sitting/lying position.

Being so far from home, I have no one to relieve me for a break, I have no other family here. The other moms I know from the pain clinic who live in the area are supportive. They bring things for Alex to do to try to keep her mind off her misery. They bring us food. They visit frequently. I don't know what I would do without them, but Alex doesn't want me to leave her with them or with anyone else for long and I feel the same way. Where would I go if I left the hospital anyway? I don't have a car and I don't know the area. Showering is difficult because I have to find a time when I can leave the room to get to a parent shower in the hallway and get dressed.

Before I find the opportunity to change out of my night-clothes, Alex's nurse tells me that the doctor needs to talk to me. He is waiting so I need to come right away. Why can't he come to Alex's room as he always does? This is unusual.

I follow the nurse down the hall past the nurses' station and into a room with four doctors sitting in chairs in a sort of semicircle—three men and one woman. What is this about? I notice Alex's attending physician and her new psychologist right away. They are the only doctors I recognize. The attending watches me intently as I enter the room. The other doctors don't make eye contact, almost as if they feel uncomfortable for me, coming to a meeting in my nightclothes. Everyone in the room wears a serious expression. The attending asks me to sit down and I do, shortly after he stands, taking a position of power.

Alex's attending is clearly in charge. Everyone introduces him or herself. The woman, a psychologist, is the superior of the psychologist who met with Alex. Maybe he is her resident. The attending goes on to tell me that the group has decided that Alex should be transferred to the psych ward. What? Are they out of their minds? He says that based on their observations and the psychologist's judgment, they feel confident that Alex suffers from conversion disorder. They have already spoken with the attending in the psych ward and they will accept her.

I can't believe it. Are they really going to commit Alex to the psych ward? Can they do that against my will? Here I am, sitting with them in my pajamas no less, and they are telling me that my daughter is crazy. I panic—then I cry. I feel so mad at myself for crying but I just can't help it. This is so unfair! How can they blindside me like this? I'm not prepared for this discussion. Then it dawns on me. They knew I wouldn't be prepared for the discussion. They wanted it that way. As that realization dawns, I can almost feel a transformation taking shape within me. I begin to feel like the Incredible Hulk. My back straightens, my shoulders lift. I can breathe deeply again without the short hiccups from crying. Oh, there will be no more crying. The tears are gone, they are replaced with strength and determination. How dare they treat me this way! How dare they dismiss Alex's issues as being in her head! This is not okay. Alex needs Resilience, Strength, and Determination to beat RSD and now I need it to protect her. Damn it. If that's what I need, I'm ready.

Bring it on . . . .

I begin spewing questions.

"What qualifies a resident to determine Alex has conversion disorder after just a few visits with her? What background work have you done in making this diagnosis? Have you even spoken to the psychologist from the pain clinic?" The pain clinic is part of the same hospital system and Alex had been there for months. I know he hasn't spoken to her because I did. She is on our side with this. I learn later that the attending (the director of the pain clinic) had been in contact with the psychologist at the pain clinic who actually said that she did not believe that there was enough information for a diagnosis of conversion disorder. So he knows that she disagrees as well.

I am on a roll. I don't even pause between questions for them to respond. I no longer care what they have to say. "I need some clarification, isn't conversion disorder a diagnosis of exclusion, meaning it is only a diagnosis if other diagnoses, often neurological diseases, are ruled out? As far as I know we haven't had an examination by a neurologist. Am I mistaken?" I pause now, but only because I know this answer with certainty.

The attending is speechless. This meeting has clearly not gone the way he planned. I figure I better stop before I start doing damage. So far, I have been respectful with an edge in my voice. I am very close to being disrespectful. I know how to argue and I can be pretty tough on people if I choose. I am smart and quick in conversations. I know it is time to get away from this one, because I am just too angry. I ask, "How can you possibly make this diagnosis when a neurologist hasn't even seen Alex during all her time at this hospital? I need time to think about what you've said but at the same time, I hope you will take what I said very seriously." I dismiss myself and go back to Alex.

A very important shift has occurred. The showdown puts me completely behind Alex. These doctors cannot be right. All my uncertainty vanishes. As I walk back to Alex's room, I feel like a weight is lifting from my shoulders. Alex and I are in this together. No secrets. No questions. I go back to Alex and I tell my eleven-year-old daughter about everything that just transpired. Her response shocks me. Alex says that she is afraid but she will go to the psych ward if it will make her better. I ask her if she wants me to check it out and she says yes. My daughter awes me.

Tuesday, May 26, 2009

Dear Journal,

They think I have conversion again. It is not a bad thing, better than everything else. But I still think it is something else but I have to believe to get better.

—Alex

The mom of the other child receives similar treatment. We both go to check out the psych ward. It seems okay but it seems to be designed for children older than ours. I have never been inside a psych ward before. It is strange. There are small dorm-like rooms, each with two beds and not much else. There is a kitchen with a large table, a bathroom off the hallway, a TV area with a couch in front of it, and a game room but without many games. It looks pretty boring. The entire place seems to be designed for teenagers. As we tour the facility, the counselor tells us how patients earn privileges by eating their food and behaving well. She says that patients don't have access to anything that could be used as a weapon to hurt themselves or others. It seems to cater to children with eating disorders, with self-destructive tendencies, with suicidal thoughts. It isn't for our children. We will not leave our children here. We are both certain of this. It feels good to be certain of something.

Juli

I am a strong woman. I've always been strong—emotional, but strong. I'm also competitive. I like to be the very best I can be at everything I do. As a teenager I figure skated competitively; as a young adult I raced Hobie Cats, small catamaran sailboats. I skippered the boat—a position often taken by the man, which just made me want to do it more, and better. I competed in nationals against men. I didn't win but I did the best I could and pushed myself hard.

I am hard on myself, expecting total effort all the time. I never give up. I am only five feet tall but people often don't realize it. I have long, dark, wavy hair and brown eyes just like Alex. I am forever on a diet—I never give up on that either. I am not fat but I am overweight, hovering around 140 pounds. I just want to be better than I am. Those qualities carry over to my parenting. They end up being some of my most important contributions to Alex's well-being.

I majored in both mathematics and education in college and became a teacher at the age of twenty-one. Before I turned thirty, I received my doctorate and taught mathematics education at a university. I love what I do and I think I am good at it. My career is important to me. Throughout Alex's illness, I continue to work. Sometimes that means keeping up with my students via email and Skype and writing books and papers by Alex's hospital bedside late into the night. My focus on work helps me through very difficult periods. It also reminds me I am a professional too, enabling me to interact with the doctors on more equal footing than most. When Alex jokes about how

I behave with the doctors, I respond, "Hey. I'm a doctor too!" So what if I'm not a medical doctor.

Finding an Ally

Interestingly, a neurologist comes to see us shortly after "the meeting." He asks Alex so many questions. He seems to really listen to her. She trusts him, which, by this time, is pretty unusual. We discuss the morning's meeting. Alex tells this neurologist that the doctors think she should go to the psych ward.

He says, "What do you think about that?" What a nice change to have a doctor ask for Alex's perspective. What she says in return almost brings him to tears.

She says, "I've been racking my brain all day to try to come up with a reason I would want to be this way. I can't come up with one. If going to the psych ward will fix me then I'll go. I don't want to go but I want to be better."

"I don't think you have conversion disorder. What I do think is that you're a very, very smart, strong young lady. I think you might have dystonia, but I'm not sure. I'm not an expert in that area. I think you need to see a neurologist who is." He turns to me and says, "I need to spend more time on this case and I will prepare a report. Your daughter is not going to go to the psych ward."

I have so many questions for him. He says that he has not seen her case before today and it is complicated and deserves more time. He says that movement disorders aren't his specialty. Movement disorders? Dystonia? I haven't heard either label before. These are things we need to investigate, but not at this hospital. They have lost my trust.

After reading the neurologist's report, the attending begins treating Alex differently. He seems to start looking for other treatment options again. The psych ward is also now off-limits.

Just after my visit there, the H1N1 virus breaks out and they are not able to accept any new patients. At least we don't have to worry about Alex being admitted against our will.

The attending says that he thinks Botox injections might help Alex's ankle. I am a little surprised I am even acknowledging him, let alone taking his suggestions after the meeting. However, I still believe he wants to help. I just don't think that what he did was helpful. It almost seems like when he can't "fix" the kids at the clinic, his next step is to decide they have conversion disorder. I think he gives up too easily.

We try the Botox. Alex is put under general anesthesia again and receives Botox injections from her toe to her hip. We feel hopeful, but once again, she experiences no change. We have to deal with where we are at this point. Alex has a severely pointed toe and her hip dislocates when she walks. She falls occasionally. It isn't safe. The attending suggests we get a brace—or AFO (ankle-foot orthotic)—for her ankle and forearm crutches to help with her stability. We also discuss building up the sole of her left shoe about an inch and a half to counteract the way she stands on her tiptoe of her right foot so her hips will be in alignment as she continues to grow. We also acknowledge the need to get a wheelchair to use for long distances to protect Alex's hip from further degeneration. We had gotten rid of the wheelchair when Alex entered the clinic the year before. This is not the path we planned to take. Buying a wheelchair rather than renting one seems so much more permanent. How can things keep getting worse?

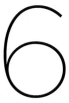

Picking Up the Pieces

As disappointed as I feel with the outcome of our trip, Alex feels even more so. As the technician fits Alex for her own wheelchair I can see her shoulders begin to sag—she feels defeated. We watch a disabled veteran come to the store in a wheelchair with camouflage paint. He needs a wheel adjusted. We see a caregiver come by to drop off a walker. Wheelchairs line the perimeter of the store and canes and walkers hang on the walls. There are all sorts of choices for finishes for canes and wheelchairs. This is a store for people who are permanently disabled. Will Alex be permanently physically disabled? It sure seems like it. Otherwise, why do we need to buy a wheelchair? Even the wheelchair has to be special. We need one light enough that she can wheel it around. Her joints are so loose we don't want to damage anything else, like her shoulders, by using the wheelchair. I need to be able to lift it up into my minivan. At five feet tall, that is not easy. She chooses a metallic blue model. At least she tries to think about style. She now has to use forearm crutches to get around; a big, cumbersome sneaker for her left foot to raise it an extra inch and a half; and an AFO for her right ankle. We hope the AFO will keep her from breaking her ankle again while her foot remains in that severely pointed position. On top of all this, she starts middle school in a few months. She needs help.

We find that help in a surfer from Cocoa Beach, Florida. After returning from the hospital in New England, we learn of another girl who had not had a great experience at this same hospital. She also has RSD and her family, in search of a cure went to the best place they could find. She eventually began working with a psychologist in Cocoa Beach after her return from New England without improvement. This psychologist got her to walk again. Marc speaks to her mother and she has nothing but good things to say about this doctor. Our daughters' situations are somewhat different but Marc and I decide to set up an appointment with this doctor just the same.

His Cocoa Beach office is more than an hour from our home but finding a psychologist smart enough to work with Alex proves challenging. We tried several after the worry-tree incident, as Alex's issues are far too complex to pin them to the worry tree in her mind, as that crazy psychologist many years ago suggested. That is how we ended up going to the good one in Gainesville, but he is even farther away. We need someone we can get to regularly who will see through Alex's barriers and instill the fight back in her. She will need it.

We find all of this and more in this psychologist. He understands pain, having endured a shark attack while surfing that took part of his foot. He has been through several leg surgeries and still surfs. Alex connects with him immediately. He is calm, cool, and intelligent, and he knows how to listen and get Alex to open up. Even the view out his office window is calming. He is on the fifth floor of a building and his window looks out over the rolling waves of the Atlantic Ocean.

This doctor uses hypnosis along with more mainstream methods to help Alex to believe in herself again. The transformation amazes us. Her physical state stagnates but her mental state makes leaps and bounds from where it was while she was in the hospital. She develops a "Yes I Can" attitude. While we can't find a way to help her get back to the life she had before she got sick, we can help her to live where she is.

We also find a Pilates instructor with a studio near Cocoa Beach. She works with Alex each week to help with strengthening and stretching. She understands Alex as she suffers from cervical dystonia. It seems we needed to find people who have withstood hardship to understand Alex's needs to be able to push her without grinding her down.

By the end of the summer, Alex is ready to begin middle school, using a wheelchair a majority of the time. She wears a white plastic brace with a Scooby Doo cartoon embedded in the back and molded to her pointed foot (her AFO). It provides a bit of a contrast to the young lady she is becoming. She is almost as tall as me now. She wears one sneaker with a sole an inch and a half thick. This makes her taller than me. She rarely wears pants due to her leg pain. And she uses forearm crutches when not in her wheelchair, only for short distances and inside the house. Not the most ideal conditions to begin middle school.

Surviving Middle School

Alex's middle school serves about 1,400 students in four main buildings, three of them two stories tall. Only one houses an elevator. The second floors of the other buildings are connected to that building by outdoor breezeways that are not conducive to transit in a wheelchair and much too large for Alex to negotiate on forearm crutches. We purchase a wheelchair backpack for her to be able to carry her own things. With extra time, we feel she can get from one class to another on her own, until we learn that the doors around campus don't have handicapped-access door openers—those round buttons you press to make the door open automatically. We are shocked. The school is only a few years old. How could it have been built with such poor wheelchair accessibility? Alex will need assistance to get from one class to the next. Still, Alex keeps a good attitude until the first day of school.

The worst thing you can possibly be as a brand-new sixth grader in middle school is different. The second worst thing you can be is partnered with someone different. The school's plan to overcome the lack of accessibility in the school is to ask Alex's classmates to bring her from class to class. She is in all gifted classes, art, and band. Surely other gifted students will have similar schedules. The teachers ask for volunteers to help Alex in each class. No one volunteers. The children aren't mean or malicious. They don't pick on Alex. They just don't choose to be with the different kid. They are still learning their own way around. While it has nothing to do with Alex, Alex feels as if it does. She feels like an outcast.

In every class all day on this miserable first day of school, her teachers do the same thing. They ask for volunteers to work with Alex in class, they ask for volunteers to bring her to the next class. Alex waits through the awful silence while the other students busy themselves not volunteering. I can't even begin to fathom how uncomfortable that must be for all involved—but especially for Alex.

Alex feels so relieved when she gets to lunchtime. Now she can be with her eight friends from elementary school, the kids who choose to stick by her. It is unfortunate that their schedules don't match hers because they would have helped her get from class to class. When she recounts her lunch experience at the end of the day our entire family has a good laugh. When she gets to the cashier to pay for her food, the lunch lady signs to her. She doesn't sign to any of the other students, just Alex. Does she assume that Alex can't hear because she can't walk? Alex had taught herself sign language almost two years earlier. I don't even remember what prompted her to learn sign language. She doesn't want to embarrass the lunch lady so she just signs back. This continues throughout Alex's entire stay in sixth grade.

Alex eventually finds her niche in middle school. The school ultimately uses the assistance of an aide, Miss Sue, to bring Alex between classes. Alex and Miss Sue form a strong bond. Alex confides in Sue during the school day. She tells Sue when her pain is particularly bad. She discusses her fears and what makes her happy. Sue speaks with Alex as a friend but in a motherly way. She keeps in constant communication with me as well, letting me know when Alex has good days and bad.

Alex begins playing flute in band. Everyone is sitting during band. Alex fits in. We add private flute lessons to the piano lessons after school so she will do well in band.

Alex also joins Odyssey of the Mind, a problem-solving club where students form and work in teams to solve problems in creative ways. They spend a good part of the school year working on a given task and then compete against other teams while judges critique their performance. Alex enjoys the club and her team members. They accept her disability and work together beautifully. Their task includes making a vehicle to transport team members as part of a skit. The group works to make a contraption to allow Alex to sit in the center with other students pushing and peddling. It is built upon an old tricycle. Another part of the challenge is to keep all expenditures under $150. Including Alex involves effort and her six other team members happily step up.

One aspect of Odyssey of the Mind competitions involves spontaneous challenges. With these challenges, the team is given a prompt and they need to come up with creative oral responses to the prompt within a limited amount of time. At one of the county competition practice sessions, Alex's team is asked, "What is the last thing you want to hear your surgeon say as you're going under for surgery?" With a straight face, sitting in her wheelchair with her leg in a brace in front of all the other teams and coaches, Alex says, "Now which leg is it?"

As part of the gifted social studies curriculum, the students are required to complete a National History Day project, choosing a historical occurrence that had a major impact. Alex chooses to research and present the Americans with Disabilities Act (ADA). She feels it might be a good way to help people in her school understand her situation and the need to make the school more accessible. Determined to experience life to the best of her ability, she wants nothing to hold her back.

Living in the "Now" while Looking for Answers

It is October 3, 2009, and it is Alex's twelfth birthday. She is swimming with dolphins at Discovery Cove. She needs her wheelchair to get around the park and we need to carry her into the water but she does it. She says it is the best day of her life.

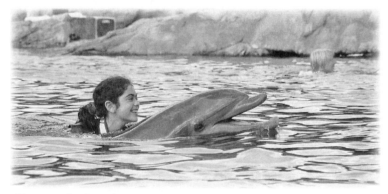

Alex, on the best day ever.

Alex does her best to live as she is but she isn't satisfied. The pain in her back seems to be resolving itself and the pain in her knee is far better but her foot gets more and more pointed, if that is even possible. The lift in her shoe has to be made taller to keep her hips level. Alex lives but she wants to live better; she wants to get better. She asks me not to stop looking for help; that is all I need to hear. Have I become too accepting of Alex's condition? I renew my efforts to find a cure. I write a letter that I send to anyone and everyone I can think of contacting. My university is in the process of starting a medical school. I send the letter to the president and provost of my university in case they have useful contacts through their efforts with the medical school. Here is a portion of the letter:

Friday, November 20, 2009
To Whom It May Concern:

We are sending this letter in search of ideas and answers. Our daughter, Alex, is in a wheelchair. She cannot walk and we don't know why. On the way to school the other day, she said, "I like that we don't have eight doctors appointments every week anymore, don't get me wrong; I just want to be sure we are still looking for a way to fix this." What follows is in response to that plea. Here is Alex's story:

Alex has seen many doctors, including pediatricians, neurologists, orthopedists, rheumatologists, anesthesiologist, psychologists, and psychiatrists. Alex works out almost every day in Pilates, our home gym, or our swimming pool in an effort to regain strength and mobility. Her strength is increasing while her mobility is decreasing. She receives psychological support that includes hypnosis once per week. Alex is supervised by a psychiatrist although she is not on psychiatric medications. She does take Trileptal, Zanaflex, and Celebrex twice daily. She gets extremely drowsy after she takes the medication and wishes she could take less. However, she is still in considerable pain and her hip continues to spasm so we have not reduced her medication.

Yet, in spite of all this, Alex is a remarkable twelve-year-old girl (see her picture below) with a terrific sense of humor, a caring character, and a quick mind. She is making almost straight A's in her coursework, which consists of all gifted classes. She is very frustrated by her current condition. She is hoping, as are we all, that she will find a way to overcome her disability and walk this year. In Alex's words, "When I grew up, I wanted to be a vet; I don't think it will be possible in a wheelchair. So I've been thinking about different possibilities I could be when I get older that you can do in a wheelchair but I still really want to be a vet. I'm hoping we can find a way to get me out of this wheelchair." Please let us know how we might facilitate your efforts in supporting Alex with these goals.

Regards,
Juli and Marc Dixon,
Alex's parents

The letter brings some attention and more questions. Based on this response, Alex's pediatrician begins to compile another letter with supporting documentation that will provide Alex's medical story in a way that I am not capable of providing. This document takes hours and hours to complete. She compiles it over the next two months. It is a labor of love. It will prove to be invaluable later.

The provost of my university sends the letter on to a pediatric neurosurgeon in Orlando. He contacts Alex's pediatrician and learns about Alex's case through the packet she compiled.

In the meantime, Alex continues to go about her life. Our family even goes on a cruise with my parents, my sister Marni, her husband, and their daughter to celebrate my parents' fiftieth wedding anniversary. We do our best to continue living.

7

Another Setback

The cruise ship is huge! I had only been on one when Alex was very young and it wasn't nearly the size of this ship. It takes quite a bit of time to check in and go through security. We are finally on board. We have our room assignment and we are heading to our room. Marc and Jessica are ahead of us. I am pushing Alex. It is difficult to navigate on the carpet and through the crowd. Jessica runs back to us.

"The room is so cool! My bed folds down from the wall and it has a ladder and Grandma and Grandpa's room is right next door. I love it!"

"Fantastic! Show us where it is." We finally get there. I can't wait to get out of the crowded hallway. Jessica uses the key and holds the door open for us.

"Mom, stop!"

"What's the matter, Alex?"

"You're smashing my wheelchair against the door."

"Sorry, I need to back up and come in straighter."

"Mom, I don't fit."

"What do you mean you don't fit? This room is handicap accessible. How can your wheelchair not fit through the door?

We have to change rooms. Let's go to the concierge." We go back to the main lobby and wait in a line that is ridiculously long. People in front of us are complaining about such minor things. I'm sure they can fit inside their staterooms. I want to cut in front of them but I control myself. It is finally our turn.

"We need a different stateroom. We were supposed to have a handicap-accessible room and my daughter's wheelchair doesn't fit through the door."

"I'm sorry, we don't have any other rooms. We are completely booked."

"What do you mean you don't have any rooms? This is unacceptable. Our reservations are for a handicap-accessible room!"

"We assigned a handicap-accessible room to your party. It is a room for three and you have four in your room. We don't have a room that can hold a family of four."

"You needed to tell us that before we got on the ship! Now what are we supposed to do?"

"You can leave the wheelchair in the hallway and we can store it when you are in the room."

"Are you kidding me? She needs her wheelchair."

"Ma'am, there is nothing we can do." The concierge is looking at the long line behind me. The other people waiting are getting impatient. I don't care. This is ludicrous.

"You have to come up with a better option."

"You can have your daughter stay in the three- person room with others in your party."

"She is a child, I cannot split her from my family! We all have to move there."

"The room is too small . . . Ma'am, you need to move aside so I can help the people behind you."

"You will move another cot into the handicap-accessible room. We will make this work."

"Fine, I will send a bellhop with a cot. Now, please move aside."

How do people live with themselves? More important, how do people with handicaps live? Life is so much more difficult and often unnecessarily so for people who are handicapped. I had no idea before all of this happened. Ignorance is probably a large part of the issue. I think that all architects, structural engineers, educators, and service personnel should have to spend a day in a wheelchair as part of training.

We maneuver the cot into the room. It is extremely cramped but we make it work.

There isn't much for Alex to do on the cruise. Activities like miniature golf are on the level with no elevator access. Still, we make the best of it. We enjoy being around family. So much of the past two years has been in doctors' offices, hospitals, and clinics away from family.

A strange thing happens to Alex on the cruise. Her right shoulder begins to spasm just like her right hip. We are watching a show on the ship. Alex calls for my attention and points to her right shoulder. It is popping back and forth just like her hip, only she is just sitting there when it happens. The last pop leaves it out of socket and Alex has to push it back in to place. It hurts and Alex handles it, though I can see the pain in her face. Can this strange thing be spreading? The other child from the clinic dealt with the same issue but in both arms. What is going on with these girls?

When we get home from the cruise, Alex's shoulder begins to pop more and more frequently. When it starts to pop, Alex removes herself from whatever situation she is in to try to take calming breaths to get it to stop. It stops after several seconds. She might be eating dinner and then her shoulder suddenly starts popping forward and back. I don't know what to do; I watch helplessly as her muscles pull her shoulder out of socket and back in again in rapid succession. It happens so frequently that Alex begins to take it in stride. I do not.

We bring Alex to a very well-respected orthopedic doctor who has been seeing her since she first got sick. We explain what is going on and it happens while we are there. He leaves the examining room and returns with a nurse. I'm curious why he needs her until I realize he wants a witness to what he is about to say. He says, "She is doing this of her own volition."

"What does that mean? You think she's doing this on purpose? Why would she want to do that? How could she even make herself do it?"

"It is like schizophrenics. They don't mean to or want to be how they are either but it is still volitional."

"Are you kidding me? I absolutely disagree with you. If you don't know what's wrong, you should just admit it rather than saying it is on purpose. You're wrong. We're done here." The doctor just stares at me; so does the nurse. I don't think they expect me to fight back. They should have been at the meeting in New England. Alex remains stoic throughout the entire exchange. We leave the office and go to the car. As soon as we get back in the car, Alex lets loose. She actually calls the doctor an ass. We still don't swear much at home but this time Alex uses proper grammar when she swears and I feel proud in some sick way. She lets off steam and I drive her back to middle school. This is where we are. Life must go on. Nothing will stop Alex from living. Or at least that's what we think.

One month later, while in band at school, her right foot becomes even more contorted. It sort of moves into a C position and turns upside down. I get a call from the school that I should come get her. She almost never calls for me to get her.

I know it is serious. When I pick her up, I can't believe what I see. What her foot is doing should not be possible. She is in terrible pain. I bring her straight to her pediatrician's office. Dr. Conway says we should go home and pack; Alex will likely need to be admitted into the hospital. She will make some calls.

They admit Alex in Orlando by evening. It is January 2010, almost two years after the last time Alex was admitted to this same hospital with pneumonia. This time she arrives in a wheelchair. With her foot in this condition, she can no longer walk, not even with her forearm crutches. She has her own hospital room. It is small but it is hers. Her wheelchair will not fit through the bathroom door. I have to carry her onto the toilet. How can this be? A hospital! I guess hospital administrators also need the training where they spend a day in a wheelchair trying to use a restroom into which they can't fit.

When the doctors examine Alex, they say they have never seen anything like it. They don't know what to do other than to give her more medication. They add Valium to her other medications. It does nothing for the pain. She can hardly bear it. I lie in her bed with her at night, holding her to help her fall asleep. I can feel her hip and shoulder spasm while she sleeps. How could anyone ever have called this conversion disorder?

We stay in the hospital a few days but make no headway and Alex feels less comfortable than we believe she will be at home. We take Alex home incapacitated.

I would do anything to help her to feel better. I can't fix her physically so I set out to do something emotionally. Her dog died about a year before. We tried to replace him with another dog but that dog was too rambunctious for Alex. Keeping him would have been unsafe. We found a new home for him.

Alex has been researching dog breeds calm enough for her and that will not shed (my requirement). She decides on a Havanese. We can't just go out shopping for one with Alex's condition so I search online. I know that this is an awful decision but it takes Alex's mind off her pain and it gives her some sort of happiness. I will do anything to make her happy.

We find a newborn puppy online. The photo looks adorable. I call the breeder who lives on the west coast of Florida. I describe our situation and ask if she thinks this puppy will be a good idea. As it turns out, the breeder is also in a wheelchair from scoliosis. She feels that a different puppy in the litter will be best for Alex—more gentle. We go with her choice. Marc thinks this a terrible idea but there is no stopping me. Alex is in love. Panda will be ready to come home to her in February.

Even the idea of getting a new puppy only takes some of the pain away. Alex can't do much of anything but stare at the pictures of her puppy that the breeder emailed. We don't know what else to do. How can things get any worse?

The Second Opinion

Eventually, Alex grows accustomed to this pain as well. It is amazing what a body can adjust to when there is no other choice. Her foot stays in the new contorted position; still grossly pointed, curved in a C position with the bottom of her foot facing up. She is not well enough to return to school. Alex can no longer wear her brace or shoe. Neither is necessary, as she can no longer walk. We have to bring the wheelchair into the house. We have never done that before. It is a sign of defeat.

We get a call from the Orlando pediatric neurosurgeon. After reading our letter and our pediatrician's packet, he has an idea of how to help Alex. He has spent time with Alex's pediatrician at her office and he has gone over Alex's files. How amazing for a neurosurgeon to put so much time into a patient he has never even seen! He says he would like us to see his mentor for a second opinion regarding his ideas. Just hearing that this doctor has a mentor impresses me, especially since he, himself, has been in practice for quite some time. Dr. Patel contacts his mentor and his mentor agrees to see us as soon as we can get to him. His mentor is located in Wisconsin. It is Friday and we set the appointment for Monday morning. We buy plane tickets to fly several hours to see yet another well-known doctor. Doing things like this is beginning to feel normal. I am amazed by what can feel normal.

The day before we leave, Alex competes in the county-level National History Day competition with her Americans with Disabilities Act project. She feels so much pain but she wants to do this. It is unusual for a sixth grader to make it to the county level. She is among a handful of sixth through eighth graders representing her school. I bring her to the competition in her wheelchair with her shoulder popping and her foot contorted.

While waiting in line at the registration area, Alex's shoulder starts popping. There is just too much stimulus. Alex says, "Wheel me into the bathroom. I need to get out of here." I do. After a few minutes, her shoulder stops and we return to register.

The competition is at a middle school. The students go into classrooms where their project boards are on display. They go into the rooms on their own. Parents and other students wait outside while the students make their presentations to three judges. I hate to send Alex in without me. What if her shoulder starts popping? Alex says she will be fine and I stay in the hall peeking through the little window in the classroom door. I can see the backs of the judges but I can't see Alex. They are standing in front of Alex's presentation board while Alex sits next to it in her wheelchair explaining her project.

She makes it through the presentation, but just barely.

"How did you do?"

"Okay . . . one of the judges asked me why I wasn't smiling. She said I should feel proud of myself for making it to the county competition. I told her that my shoulder had been dislocating the whole time and it was difficult to smile when you are in as much pain as I am."

"Oh, Alex, I can't believe you said that . . . what did she say?"

"She didn't know what to say but it felt good to tell her."

I don't think many people realize what Alex endures on a daily basis. Alex qualifies for the state-level National History Day competition with her foot pointed, upside down, and curved in a C and her shoulder dislocating. The state competition is scheduled for May in Tallahassee, Florida. Alex is looking forward to the trip. I feel so proud of her for making it through the competition with all she has to handle.

We head to Wisconsin to see a world-renowned neurosurgeon. He will know what to do to help Alex.

PART II:
THE UNIMAGINABLE

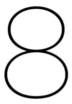

A Bumpy Start

Alex, Marc, and I are off to Wisconsin to see a pediatric neurosurgeon. Between her pain and not being able to walk, it is difficult to travel with Alex. We use her wheelchair to get her on the plane, then check it at the gate. Alex sits next to the window watching the luggage being loaded onto the plane. While she looks on, her wheelchair comes down from the gate. She watches as the baggage handler throws her wheelchair onto the conveyer to send it into the plane. It teeters on the edge of the conveyor then crashes to the ground just as it is to go into the plane. We can't believe it. It just rolls off, falls to the ground, and bounces. We know it is badly damaged. Alex begins to panic. How will she get off the plane? How will she get to the hospital to meet with the doctor? She is now completely dependent on her chair. It amazes me that the baggage handler isn't more careful.

As soon as I see what has happened, I report the incident to the flight attendant. She passes on the information to the baggage handler's supervisor. The supervisor happens to have a prosthetic leg. He is wearing shorts and we can see a metal bar where a leg should be. We watch through the little airplane window as the supervisor, one hand on his hip and the other jabbing the air in front of the baggage handler's face, screams at the baggage handler. It looks like a cartoon show on TV where one character yells at the other and the other's hair flies straight back from the hot air being blown out in anger. That helps to lighten our mood but it doesn't help us with our new problem. We are spending twenty hours in another state far from home where we know no one and now Alex's wheelchair is broken.

After we land, we take off the handles from our luggage and use them as straps to rig the wheelchair to work in an attempt to correct its newly twisted form. It needs to be fixed but that will have to wait until we return to Orlando, as we won't be in town long enough. At least that is what we think.

Extending Our Stay

The pediatric neurosurgeon is kind. He asks many questions and takes time to make sense of Alex's condition. I had sent the file her pediatrician had compiled in preparation for our visit. The doctor says it is the best letter from a doctor he has ever seen—more like a small notebook than a letter. Alex has been through so much by the time we get here that telling about it is no small undertaking. Reading about it isn't either. Clearly this doctor does his homework.

After examining Alex, the doctor suggests we stay here so he can do an extended baclofen test. He thinks baclofen is the best option to get Alex's hip to stop spasming. That is what he calls what we describe as her hip popping. We originally came to see him because of her ankle and foot. He isn't sure the baclofen will loosen her ankle but he thinks the hip spasms are a bigger issue.

We tell him we already tried intrathecal baclofen but he does it differently. He suggests he surgically place a port in Alex's abdomen that connects to her spine so he can perform a continuous intrathecal baclofen test. This way, the dose can continue to be increased over a six- to ten-day period to see if there is a point where the baclofen will help. The port will remain after the test if it isn't helpful and it will be replaced with a pump if the test is successful. Hold on, he is going to leave the thing inside my daughter? Is he serious?

He is and it is our best option. He has used this procedure many times with children with cerebral palsy. It is one of his specialties. Once again, we are out of options. We decide to go through with it.

Here we are in snowy Wisconsin with a return flight to Orlando scheduled for four hours from now and a plan to admit Alex to the hospital tomorrow morning. We have so much to do. At least we will have time to have Alex's wheelchair fixed, courtesy of the airline. We arrange for it to be picked up from the hospital when we are admitted tomorrow. We have no car, no extra clothes, and no place to stay. We cancel our flight and contact the Ronald McDonald House.

You hear so many stories about how the Ronald McDonald House helps people. Well, here is another one. There is no room at the House because it is being renovated but they arrange for a handicap-accessible room at a participating hotel. A volunteer driver from the Ronald McDonald House picks us up at the hospital, takes us to a department store, and waits for us to buy clothes and other provisions. He brings us right to our hotel. He is a retired economics professor who volunteers at the House each week doing whatever is needed. He makes just the right amount of small talk for us to feel comfortable. He even tells us about the area as we drive. When we get to the store, he tells us to take as much time as we need in the store; he has a book to read and will be fine. He is great.

Once at the hotel, Alex feels so worried. She is in pain, afraid, and so sad. She likes to draw to relax herself. She is quite good at it. She draws a picture of her new puppy. It is February

7. Her puppy will be ready to come home in two weeks. I feel so glad her dog provides some comfort even though she has never even held him.

The Baclofen Test

The surgery to place the port goes fine. The doctor asks Alex what she wants to dream about as she is going under and she says Panda. Again, I feel thankful for having gone ahead with purchasing the puppy online. Recovery is difficult. Alex has to lie flat on her back for two full days to avoid a spinal headache. After that she begins to rise up toward a sitting position very slowly. The baclofen is increased over the next week.

Alex has a few issues after the surgery. She feels sick to her stomach and she won't eat. I finally get her to eat a little but she just vomits everywhere. She also can't pee. We try everything. We try every size and shape bedpan in the hospital. We put her hand in warm water; we pour water right over her. We even put peppermint oil in her bedpan—don't ask me why, but someone suggests it so we do it. Nothing works. It is time to catheterize her. She hasn't peed in more than twenty-four hours. Nobody can catheterize her successfully. I feel so bad for Alex. Here she is, twelve years old with nurse after nurse, both female and male trying to catheterize her. The neonatal ICU nurse is finally successful. What a relief, but why can't she pee?

I try to keep a positive face for Alex. I use email as my outlet to other adults. I share simple updates, things that make me worried, and things that make me hopeful. So many people are worried about Alex: our family, her teachers, our friends from home, the friends we made at the clinic in New England, my coworkers—the list goes on. Once again we are far from our home and support network. I send these email updates to all of those people. It is a fairly long and diverse list. I continue to send these emails during most of our stay in this hospital.

Wednesday, February 10, 2010 5:10 PM

Alex made it through surgery well. She now has a port in her abdomen connected to her spine. She has incisions in both her back and abdomen and is in pain and generally miserable. We will wait to see if the baclofen being introduced through the port connected to her spine works on her spasms. If it does, then we will schedule the next surgery here and we will start the process over again. The next surgery will entail placing a permanent baclofen pump where the port is and cutting the Achilles tendon in her foot to release the contracture that the surgery yesterday indicated is now fixed. If the procedure we are doing now doesn't work, then I don't have a clue as to what is next. Let's just hope it works.

—Juli

The doctor keeps checking in to see if the baclofen is working but it isn't doing anything. Every time he comes to visit, he asks Alex if she has any questions. She always has questions. He gives her three questions per visit. Her questions are pretty impressive. She asks how the baclofen works, why she has spasms, what causes spinal headaches—all sorts of questions—and Dr. Alden answers them all.

This goes on for six days. Alex cannot eat much of anything. She has a catheter to pee. Her baclofen is being raised substantially, and there is no change. At night I stay with Alex in her hospital room and Marc stays at the Ronald McDonald House. Marc can't stay with us indefinitely. Jessica is at home with my parents. I have someone covering my classes at the university, but Marc needs to get back to work. Life is going on without us back home. Alex just missed her Odyssey of the Mind competition. She is sad when she hears that she missed the competition but she is proud of her group. They worked so hard all year.

Sunday, February 14, 2010 10:14 AM
Hi Juli,

Alex's Odyssey team took 3rd place. We dedicated the performance to Alex. Then they did an "all hands in 1-2-3-Alex" before they started. It made my heart sing! They are going to go on to compete at the State competition on April 10. We have a few things to polish. Hopefully Alex will be able to go. She was certainly there in spirit yesterday!

—Ms. Poarch

It is Valentine's Day. As Marc is walking to the hospital from the Ronald McDonald House to say good-bye to us, a custodian from Alex's hospital wing reminds him to give me a valentine. That is so far from our minds it is almost funny, but not really. Alex is the only one who makes a valentine. She has to make it while in a reclined position because she is still not able to sit all the way up. She gives it to Marc before he leaves. Marc catches a flight home. I hate for him to go. Alex just doesn't seem to be doing well. She has lost so much weight. Her foot is still contorted. She isn't able to pee. Things are just bad.

Out of Control

About five hours after Marc leaves, Alex's spasms change. It is different from before. They are no longer isolated to her hip and shoulder. They take over the entire right side of her body. They frighten her and they frighten me as well.

I call the nurse in to take a look. The nurses at this hospital are outstanding—patient, kind, and knowledgeable. They work so hard to help Alex.

The nurse sees one of the spasms and contacts the resident to let him know of Alex's change. The resident must not think it is anything to worry about because he doesn't come immediately. When he does come, he doesn't seem alarmed. I calm down a little.

The calm doesn't last long. The new spasms increase in intensity, frequency, and duration throughout the entire day. By the time Marc gets home from the airport, I call him to tell him how scared I am. I don't know what to do. The entire right side of Alex's body flails around for about twenty seconds every twenty minutes or so. Her hand smashes into her face, her leg crashes against the bed, and her hip and shoulder repeatedly dislocate during the entire episode. Her eyes roll up in her head and she blacks out for a few seconds. Then she makes this awful choking sound and it is over.

I think the nurses feel scared as well. By evening we have a nurse in the room with us nonstop. The nurses rearrange their coverage of other patients to do this. They are all that are keeping me together; I cannot even imagine being in the room with Alex without them. Alex's face gets sore from her hand smashing into it. Her foot hits the rails of the bed if someone isn't there to protect her. Someone needs to be next to her continuously. The nurse and I tag team to accomplish this. We put crash pads on her bed rails. Alex's spasms are beginning to look more like seizures than anything else.

Things continue to go downhill. By ten p.m. Alex is having spasms every five minutes. Her spasms are so violent that it takes two people to keep her safe. We keep calling the resident in; I want her doctor to see this. I need him to help. I can't get anyone other than the nurses to take this seriously. I cannot handle this alone. I need someone with me.

I call home and ask for help. I just can't do this on my own. My parents are still at my house. My dad says he will fly up to us on the first flight he can get. I feel so relieved. My dad is like a rock. He can handle anything. He calls back with his flight information. He will be here by tomorrow afternoon. Okay, I can make it alone with Alex until then. At least I think I can.

Alex keeps getting worse and worse. I make frantic calls home even though there is absolutely nothing anyone there can do. I just have to hear their voices. Marc and my parents all get on the phone every time I call. They can hear the absolute panic in my voice. They can hear Alex spasming in the background. I have to drop the phone to help Alex and then pick it up again during a break in her spasms. She spasms every one to two minutes now. I can't imagine how helpless Marc and my parents must feel, probably even more so than me. I literally think Alex will die. I tell Marc he better get back up here too.

Marc finds a flight to get him to us a few hours before Dad. I don't know how I will make it until he gets here. I have been leaning over Alex's bed helping her with the spasms for twelve straight hours. I feel tired, sore, and scared.

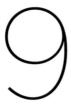

The ICU

The nurses become more concerned. By one a.m. there are often two nurses in the room with us helping at the same time. I know they have contacted the residents several times. One resident finally comes to look in again but he still won't contact the doctor. It is unbelievable to me that he doesn't think this is an emergency. Do the attending doctors put that much fear into the residents? It just doesn't make sense. I feel like shaking him.

It is two a.m. and one of the nurses just went to the other side of the floor to the ICU to ask the ICU resident to look in on Alex. I have a feeling this is not standard procedure and I am so thankful to the nurse for doing this. The ICU resident takes one look at Alex and starts the procedures for moving Alex to the ICU.

I feel partly relieved and partly more panicked. If they are moving Alex over, they must think that Alex is in trouble. I am no longer tired. Adrenaline kicks in. I am absolutely alert.

Things move fast in the ICU. Doctors are all over the place. They connect Alex to an EEG immediately. She has electrodes glued all over her head. Alex has very thick hair. This is no small undertaking. A team of doctors checks all sorts of things. The number of monitors connected to her is overwhelming. What are they looking for? Do they think she will die? It sure seems like it.

It's Probably Psychogenic

The EEG is negative; the spasms are not seizures. A relief. But if they aren't seizures, what are they? Whatever they are, they continue to get worse. Alex hasn't slept in about twenty hours. She has been spasming for the past twelve hours or so. She can feel the spasms coming on. She says, "Oh no, here it comes again." Her eyes roll up into the back of her head and she sort of blacks out; her right leg starts smashing up and down; her right arm flails around and smashes up hard against her face. Her teeth jam hard against each other. Toward the end of the spasm—it probably lasts twenty to thirty seconds although it seems like an eternity—she makes a choking sound. Her wrist, shoulder, and hip are dislocated, and her foot is curled back to her butt. Her joints dislocate repeatedly during the entire spasm. After the spasm, she straightens herself out, which often means putting her own dislocated wrist back in place. Then she is coherent until the next spasm starts.

Her doctor's resident comes to see her after we are admitted to the ICU. He sees that her EEG is normal and has the audacity to tell me that these episodes are likely psychogenic. I turn into the Hulk immediately and say, "How dare you say they are psychogenic. We have been down that road. You are not correct; don't speak to me about that again." My reaction is instantaneous and strong. The days of questioning my daughter have been gone since the first day I turned into the Hulk—the morning I was confronted by the team of doctors while still in my nightclothes. This resident is not going to take us there again. I want nothing to do with him. I don't even like to associate him with Dr. Alden, even though I know he is Dr. Alden's resident so they are very much associated. Dr. Alden makes me feel safe and protected. This resident makes me feel uncomfortable and worried. I am angry at him for his statement—I take it more like an accusation—but deep down I know he probably just said it because he is young and inexperienced; so why do I feel this way? I push the feelings aside and move on with my role of protecting Alex.

The day continues with Alex spasming this way. The nurses check in frequently but they are not able to stay with us like the nurses had the previous day. How can Alex survive this? I feel so tired by this point, it is all I can do to keep Alex from injuring herself during the spasms.

Marc arrives by midday and my dad arrives a few hours after that. Alex's doctor stops the baclofen test. We are now beyond that. We have to stop the spasms. By nightfall, she has been spasming for a day and a half. The doctor tries various medications.

Marc, my dad, and I take turns sitting with Alex through the night. I fall asleep right in the chair in Alex's room the minute it is my turn to rest. It isn't even a reclining chair. I don't ever remember being so tired. Marc feels so afraid and stressed out, he can barely function. He just stares at Alex then turns away and cries. He can't help it. It is clear we need help but we don't know how to get it.

By morning, I feel desperate. My daughter is still spasming. I am beyond functioning. What are we going to do? Alex's pediatrician calls from Florida to check on us. I share my fear and frustration. She speaks to me as a friend and a doctor and helps me to see what we need and gives me the language to ask for it. I need so much; I don't have the tools to advocate for Alex and myself in this situation. After her call, I ask for and receive nursing support at Alex's bedside around the clock. Without her helping to empower me, who knows what would have happened. What do people do who do not have the support system I have? I am friends with Alex's pediatrician. She has my cell phone number to call me. I feel comfortable asking her for this sort of advice and she feels comfortable giving it. It is invaluable. However, it does not stop Alex's spasms.

Doctors worry about muscle breakdown from all the spasms and repeated dislocations. The challenge is to give Alex enough medication to get the spasms to stop without keeping her from breathing on her own because otherwise she will need a breathing tube. I can't even fathom how she can keep this up. However, Alex is still very much aware. She makes it very clear that she does not want a breathing tube. She knows about it from her experiences with general anesthesia and she hates it. I promise to do my best to avoid having her need to get a breathing tube. As we continue to raise her medication with no effect, it becomes a clear possibility I will not be able to keep that promise. Alex and I are a team and I don't feel as though I can keep this from her. I tell Alex and she understands. I think she has a sense of the seriousness of her condition.

All day a team of doctors works together to come up with a plan to help Alex. Her doctor even videotapes her spasming and sends the video to his colleague in another state for a consultation. I ask for a copy of the video. I don't think her doctors at home can possibly imagine it without proof. Alex has been spasming for two full days and she hasn't eaten for a week. She can't go on like this much longer but her medication cannot be raised any more without placing her under sedation, much like inducing a coma. I feel so relieved not to face this alone.

Grandpa

My dad is my rock. I have rarely seen him cry. The only time I remember seeing him cry is when my mom had just had surgery for breast cancer and my dad, my sister, and I were sitting together discussing the implications of Mom's cancer. He is not overly emotional but he is sensitive. He understands the emotions of others. He had to learn that living in a household with my mother, my sister, and me. My dad is also very intelligent. He is retired now but he was a science education professor. He still reads quite a bit and keeps his mind active by taking and teaching courses related to sailing and navigation. He even took a course in trigonometry at age seventy.

He is the perfect person to have with us at the hospital because he is so levelheaded, logical, and knowledgeable. He helps Marc and me come up with questions for the doctors and then helps us process the responses. He has been with us through Alex's entire illness, along with my mom. We are a very close family. My parents do almost everything together. For my dad to come to us, and my mom to stay with Jessica, you know they understand the seriousness of our situation.

Alex just adores my father. He has this stupid joke he always tells: What is purple and goes bang, bang, bang, bang? . . . A four-door grape. Then he laughs and laughs and laughs. It is the same way every time he tells it and he tells it frequently, mostly to my daughters and mostly because they ask him to do so. Even amid Alex's awful spasms, when she first sees my dad, she asks him to tell her the joke. And of course, he does. She has him wrapped around her finger.

10

A Coma to Save Her Life

Are you kidding me? We are going to place Alex into a coma voluntarily? Who does that? The plan—to induce a coma and begin Alex on a medication called Haldol—does not have complete consensus because of drug choice, but those who don't agree don't have other suggestions.

I stay with Alex while she has her breathing tube inserted. I feel so helpless. I think I hold my breath through the entire process. My father stays with me with his arm around me. Marc can't handle things like this. He goes down the hall and cries. He must feel so alone. At least I have my father here. We are so far away from home and from all our family and friends. It is just the four of us—Alex, Marc, my dad, and me.

Alex's spasms finally stop as the coma is induced. Now we wait. And watch. It is surreal to watch the machine breath for Alex. I feel an odd sense of relief to see her body rest.

Everyone tells me I need to rest while Alex is in her coma. I should go get some sleep. There are even beds in the sleeping rooms in the ICU. The Ronald McDonald House provides them. Each day, families of patients in the ICU sign up to get a "sleep room" for the night. There aren't enough rooms for everyone and they are coveted. The sleep rooms are in a very quiet hallway of the ICU. There is a single bed, a lamp, and a nightstand in each room. There are no monitors flashing and beeping like in the patients' rooms. There are no nurses walking in and out. They are very helpful to families. They terrify me. I can't get myself to leave Alex's room to go sleep in a bed. I can't leave her side. Marc sleeps in the sleeping room and my dad sleeps at the Ronald McDonald House. I stay in Alex's room, staring at the monitors, watching the machine breath for her, and hoping the medicine will work. It is a strange feeling; like if I can just stare at her hard enough I can will her to get better, but this is clearly not the case.

I send emails to family at all times of day and night giving updates. I think the emails are somewhat therapeutic for me. They help me to organize my thoughts relative to what is going on with Alex. Sometimes they are short updates and other times they are much more involved. I can't imagine what they are like for the people getting them.

Friday, February 19, 2010 12:28 AM

Alex has pneumonia in both lungs. Marc has completely fallen apart.

—Juli

I become addicted to the daily rounds when the attending doctors and the residents stand outside Alex's door and discuss her case. I am allowed to participate in these meetings. The doctors answer my questions and listen to my suggestions. It might be just to help me to cope with the stress; regardless, it works. I have a need to know everything about Alex's case. I keep notes and check the doctors' numbers. I'm sure I focus on insignificant bits of information but at least it gives me something to focus on.

Friday, February 19, 2010 1:01 AM

The thought is that she aspirated during her spasms when her eyes would roll up in her head and she would black out. She is so damn smart; she told us she was getting pneumonia between spasms. The good thing is that we caught it early. I told the ICU doc I was almost certain it was pneumonia. She went with that and started her on antibiotics. She also ordered an x-ray stat (Alex gets a chest x-ray every day at 4 a.m. due to the breathing tube but we didn't wait for that one). Her x-ray this morning at 4 a.m. was clear. The x-ray this evening showed bilateral, lower-lobe pneumonia. We caught this very early . . . .

More later,
Juli

We start Alex on a feeding tube while she is in her coma. Even that doesn't go easily. The doctors try several times to pass the feeding tube and it won't make it down all the way. It has to be passed using a special procedure but at least she is getting food.

The only time I leave Alex's room is to Skype with Jessica. I bring my computer out into the hallway outside Alex's room. We haven't told Jessica that Alex is in a coma or even in the ICU. We don't think Jessica needs to know. She doesn't have either of her parents to hold her to help her handle the news. We just keep telling Jessica that Alex is sleeping or that she isn't feeling well enough to Skype. We also tell her we aren't allowed to Skype in the hospital room so she is unable to see Alex. Jessica accepts this. I wonder if she knows something is up. If she does, she doesn't let on. My dad fills my mother in on the latest news during a separate phone call. My mom handles everything internally and keeps a happy face for Jessica.

It is coming up on Jessica's birthday and we are fairly certain we won't be home in time. It is surreal to go online while sitting in Alex's hospital room to order a birthday present for Jessica. Marc and I make a guilt purchase of a giant karaoke machine. We want to be sure she feels loved and has fun even though having fun seems like such a remote idea from where we are. My mom agrees to host a slumber party with eight girls. My mother is doing her best to keep Jessica's life as normal as possible in our absence. It seems so strange but crucially important for Jessica's life to go on as smoothly as possible—something we can actually control.

ABANDONED (BY JESSICA DIXON)

Mom, Alex, and Dad are leaving to fly someplace for a second opinion for a surgery. This is another "cure." They are running out of options. Even I know it and they don't tell me very much. Since Alex's foot started turning upside down every time I see her, I want to cry and I am not even the one in pain. She just lies there on our parents' bed. Her face strains with pain as she fights a battle I can't fight with her. How can people even consider she is faking? How could a young girl make her foot turn upside down? Why would she want to? It looks like the same amount of pain as the instant you break a bone except it is not just one moment, it drags on forever. Well, maybe it's worse pain than that. I don't even feel that pain, but you can easily read it on her face. I know doctors by now. If they can't fix it, they want to make it seem like it's your fault. They'd rather keep a good reputation than help a patient in pain. They are all liars. They want money not to help people who need it.

Mom, Alex, and Dad get on the plane and fly away, taking my heart with them. For some reason it feels a lot like when they flew away to go to the pain clinic, but they will be back in two days—not months like before. I am done with these stupid "experts." I've been dragged from appointment to appointment and they do nothing that ever works. Alex has gotten worse and the doctors tell us it is our fault. Yet, they are the ones who are supposed to have the answers, but guess what, THEY DON'T. Grandma and Grandpa are staying with me. They are really kind, but it seems like they don't understand. They try to look at the bright side. What is the bright side? It seems I have forgotten it.

My parents call and tell us they will be staying longer. This doctor found out what it is and will give us a cure. What do you know, maybe one doctor knows something? That is about one in twelve million. Alex can't be the only one like this. They are having a surgery and then they will come back home. Unlike the clinic, Alex could come home normal and happy. I really do miss that twinkle in her eye. I truly miss that spark of life. I asked Mom and she said they will be back in time for my birthday.

They are staying longer than I thought and my birthday is coming closer. They never have missed my birthday before. I hope they won't this year. Alex isn't feeling well and Mom and Dad say she can't talk to me. Mom and Dad set up a computer program so we can see each other. Everyone has a breaking point and I am reaching mine. I scream at them over the computer. I tell them they have more than one daughter and I need them too. I tell them that seeing each other on a stupid computer screen isn't the same and it isn't. You can't hug over a computer screen and more than anything I need them to hug me now. The mean selfish me tells them that. In my head I am officially abandoned.

When we hang up I run crying into my room and my sweet, caring, strong grandmother tries to comfort me. I hug her and start crying even more. On the really lonely days I push her away. We get into bad arguments often because I am determined to get her to leave and get my parents to come home. I really love her but she isn't the same. She is my grandmother, not my mother. She is starting to take on that role and I don't like it, not at all.

I am weak. Everything I keep inside is building up pressure. It needs to come out. I hate the doctors but I don't have one to let out my wrath on. If Mom had taken me along with her to one more appointment where the doctors called Alex a faker I would have let him have it. I would have thrown a tantrum all the two-year-olds in the world would envy. Mom didn't take me because they are away with Alex somewhere else. My parents are missing everything. They missed my field trip, losing my tooth, and another week of me growing up needing them. Imagine how much anger I let out when they tell me they will miss my birthday.

Everything is already set up. For my birthday I want my family to be there. While most fourth grade girls wish for a phone or a boyfriend, I wish to be with the people I love most, even though they don't care enough to be with me. My grandma and I plan a sleepover party. We will watch a movie and play some games. Grandpa left to help Mom and Alex up there with something. They need him more than they need me.

The party is great and I push that deeper loneliness into the back of my head, but it is still there. The movie is cute and I invited a lot of girls from school. Apparently they like it and it probably moves me up a notch in their eyes. Like I care about that type of thing. My new karaoke machine especially impresses them. I know it is some guilt present to keep my parents' child off their minds so they can pretend she is all happy. I let them know I am not over the computer.

....

Friday, February 19, 2010 9:09 PM

Things are calm (knock on wood). We will begin bringing her out of sedation tomorrow, late morning. We are getting set up for deep brain stimulation on Tuesday if necessary. Please pass it on. We are sitting in Alex's room having quiet time and Marc is doing the best I've seen.

—Juli

We keep Alex in a coma for three days as the drug is introduced. It is time to begin taking her out of the coma. It just has to work. If not, our only other option left, according to the doctor, is for Alex to get a deep brain stimulator, or DBS. She will have a wire surgically implanted deep in her brain and a battery will be implanted in her chest and connected to the wire.

The intent is for the stimulation to interrupt the spasms. We are hoping to avoid this route by using Haldol. If this drug stops the spasms, we are set. Alex's neurosurgeon, Dr. Alden, sought out opinions of other experts and discussed all the possibilities with us so we understand them clearly.

Dr. Alden

Dr. Alden provides a huge amount of support for us. He has been a surgeon for more than thirty years. He gives talks all over the world and is most known for working with children with cerebral palsy. He feels that they are God's children. Dr. Alden is a deeply religious man. He is absolutely committed to what he does. His wife, Sarah, is a pediatric neurosurgery nurse. The two of them work together and make a powerful team. They look after us so well and not just directly with Alex's care. The two of them check on me to make sure I am getting outside—I'm not. I haven't been outside in almost two weeks. They begin making me go outside for fifteen minutes every day to get fresh air. I feel so afraid to leave Alex's room, it is almost more than I can bear. However, I do it because they ask me to. I trust them completely.

Even Dr. Alden's physical presence is reassuring—tall, slim, and athletic. His hands look like a surgeon's hands. His eyes are kind and gleam with intelligence. Even with his great intelligence—or maybe because of it—he is one of the few doctors who consults with everyone around him. He asks Alex's nurses for input; he asks Marc, my dad, and me for input; and he consults with other specialists. It seems like some doctors don't think they need to speak with others, whereas Dr. Alden takes the perspective that it truly does take a village to care for a sick child. Everyone around him adores him as much as we do. He has a dry sense of humor. Before Alex's coma, she jokes with him in between her spasms when she is well enough. I think he is surprised by her wit. I am fairly certain she found a special place in his heart.

We feel so fortunate to have connected with Dr. Alden and Sarah. We ask them anything and they respond honestly and openly. We know they are doing everything in their power to help Alex. That is why we are so sad and even a bit panicked when we learn they are heading to Kenya in just six months. They are selling their home and moving there to develop a pediatric neurosurgery clinic. They plan to spend the next two to four years working and living in difficult conditions to help more of God's children. They feel it is their mission. We feel thankful they have not already gone. We need them more than words can ever express.

Spasms Return

Saturday, February 20, 2010 2:00 PM

We started taking Alex out of the "coma" three hours ago and within an hour she started spasming again every minute but much more gently because she is still sedated. She was given more Haldol and now she is out again. Even with all the sedation, her shoulder dislocated with the spasm and she was able to point to tell me to pop it back in. I couldn't get her wrist back in so it is still out. I have a feeling she will be in brain surgery no later than Tuesday and possibly earlier. This is a nightmare. I think we have a diagnosis of primary hemidystonia but that is not really a cause. We may never know the cause. We met with a genetic doc yesterday who is reviewing her "notebook" over the weekend to decide what other tests to do. Because she has a port now we can get cerebrospinal fluid (CSF) whenever needed.

I am so scared. I just can't imagine what would have happened if she had gotten this bad in Orlando. Thinking back, I can see it starting over the last few months as she began to spasm more in her sleep and as her shoulder and hip dislocated more and more often. I KNOW that if she had gotten this bad in that hospital in New England she would be in restraints in the psych ward, even though it started again while she was completely sedated. . . . We told the docs today (both the neurologist and neurosurgeon are here on a Saturday and they are videotaping the entire process) that if they are successful, they better clear their calendars because there will be a steady flow of folks coming their way from the Northeast (all the kids who weren't helped there).

—Juli

How can she still be spasming through all this? How could anyone ever have thought this was on purpose? The spasms just have to stop. The discussion around Alex having surgery to get a DBS becomes more pressing.

Sunday, February 21, 2010 8:34 AM

So she is still spasming but not very often or as hard. She is still on the breathing tube—we don't know what will happen when she is actually moving. At this point she is on a relatively low dose of Haldol and we have begun to take her off one of the sedation agents (the one that causes amnesia, unfortunately, so she will remember being held down with a breathing tube). Dr. Alden is still not comfortable removing her breathing tube as he thinks there is a good chance we will need to induce this coma-like sedation again as her spasms increase. He will be back in early this morning (after church) to check on her. I adore this man.

Marc and I were up with Alex all night. We each slept about two hours. Today will probably get worse. I have never been so tired in all of my life. . . . I KNOW we need to sleep but we really don't have a choice—it is tough to explain just how hard we work here. Alex's care is excellent but the situation is so tenuous and nobody really knows what to do. Marc, Dad, and I need to remain very active members of her minute-by-minute care to keep her safe. I could never be a nurse and I have an entirely new level of respect for them, especially ICU nurses.

So, the good news is that the Haldol might be working.

—Juli

As Alex continues to come off the sedation, it becomes clear Haldol is not a viable option. Not only are her spasms continuing but the Haldol does terrible things to her. Her eyes roll up in her head and stay there for long periods of time. Her throat seems to be stretched closed. She cannot speak. She tries to sign to us but it is no use. We can't interpret her signs. When she took it upon herself to learn sign language so many years ago, none of us joined her. I feel like a bad parent not being able to communicate with her in the only way she can. If only I had learned to sign, I might be able to help her with something. It is difficult to express just how horrible it all is. Alex seems possessed by something. She has to get off the Haldol.

So we are on to our last option. The DBS.

11

Going Ahead with the Surgery

We meet with Alex's neurosurgeon, Dr. Alden, to go over options. Typically, when exploring options, Marc and I research everything about our choices and find the best doctors in the country doing those things. We look for academic journals on the topic, read them, and understand little. What we do well is to identify the people cited repeatedly in the articles about given topics. We contact those doctors by looking them up at the universities listed in the articles they publish. More often than not, they talk or email with us and help guide us to hospitals and/or doctors with expertise in those areas. I wonder how many people follow this same approach. It seems so logical but the doctors we contact often seem genuinely surprised.

We can't do this with the DBS. We were not contemplating it before Alex started these awful spasms at the hospital. We read up on it as best we can in the hospital. Dr. Alden seems to be one of the experts but what will we do when we return to Florida? The DBS requires long-term support from doctors who are familiar with its use. Through our limited Internet searches, we can find no one in Florida who works with children with the DBS. We ask Dr. Alden about this; we discuss all the options openly. He says that we can fly Alex elsewhere for surgery but we will likely not find someone in Florida to do it. He says he will provide us with names of other top doctors who do this surgery with children. We don't feel comfortable doing that. We don't dare move Alex and we feel comfortable with Dr. Alden. We decide to go ahead with the surgery in Wisconsin.

Monday, February 22, 2010 7:13 PM

Barring any unforeseen complications (oh wait, that basically describes Alex's daily life the last two years), Alex will have brain surgery at 7:30 a.m. tomorrow morning. We anticipate the recovery to be about ten days give or take, well, we have no idea. The surgery is several hours long and we won't know anything regarding its success for several days or months. Beyond ten days or so, we will transport home (somehow). If she still needs hospitalization it will be in Jax, FL . . . .

That's it for now. Marc is being absolutely amazing. Talk about rising to an impossible challenge. Alex's eyes are now dystonic and "stuck," looking up so that they are partially rolled to the back of her head but her eyes are open for long periods of time, but not always. It is eerie. I think she can see but it is not clear. Other times her eyes look normal but very sleepy and then we know she can see. She knows what is going on but her throat is also dystonic so she can't speak easily. She speaks occasionally but very softly and she doesn't say much. Her face lights up when the doctor comes to see her. She adores him and so do I. More later.

—Juli

The Haldol is just impossible. It is like Alex's muscles are involuntarily pulling her eyes so they roll back and it is stretching her vocal cords so they don't work. It is like what her foot is doing, where it is curled in a way that seems impossible, but now it is her neck and her eyes as well. Why can't anything work out for her? Now we are heading into surgery. How can this be happening? How many times have I thought that in the last two years?

The Worst Day of Our Lives

Bringing Alex to surgery is different this time. I am always allowed to go in with her and hold her as she is put under. I am to go in with her this time as well. However, this time it is so tough for her to talk. She holds on tight but she doesn't talk much. She still tries to say Panda's name as she is going under because that's whom she will dream about, but she can hardly even say his name because of what the Haldol is doing to her.

Marc, my dad, and I are brought to a special area to wait for Alex to come out of surgery. Other families wait there too. The hospital is not just for pediatric patients, although Alex is in the pediatric ICU. This area is for everyone. Most people are clearly waiting for older patients. It is so unfair that Alex has to go through so much at such a young age.

We wait and wait. The surgery takes many hours. The surgery starts with an MRI, then Alex's skull is secured in a frame so that the placement of the deep brain stimulator will be exact. The stimulator wire is placed and then Alex has another MRI to check the accuracy of its placement. The battery is placed in Alex's chest and a shunt is used to connect the wire from the top of her brain around and down her neck to the battery. The battery is typically placed in a second surgery but we don't have the luxury to wait in Alex's case. The battery is placed at the same time so programming the DBS can commence immediately. The doctor decides to use a rechargeable battery. We will need to charge it every few weeks by placing the charger over her chest for an hour or so. While a hassle, she will not need to have surgery to replace the battery for seven to nine years as opposed to every three years for a nonrechargeable battery. That is a good thing. When the battery is replaced, it will mean surgery on her chest area, not her brain. Having brain surgery just seems so wrong.

The DBS requires a change in Alex's lifestyle. She will be limited in some ways. She can not be around large magnets. She will not be able to go through airport security like everyone else. She will even need to be careful going through the security devices at department stores and libraries as they can turn off her DBS. She cannot have an MRI on any part of her body but her head and it cannot be the strongest MRI. The list goes on. It feels strange to read the list, almost surreal. It is daunting but necessary. Alex is in surgery to have the DBS placed because we have no other options.

Once Dr. Alden is satisfied with the placement of the DBS, the incision in Alex's scalp is closed back up and Alex is brought out of anesthesia. We get a few updates during the surgery; things seem to be going well. I feel like I am holding my breath all day long. We are basically silent the entire day.

Dr. Alden finally comes in with great news. Alex's surgery went beautifully. The placement of the wire is just perfect. The shunt was very difficult to pass to connect the wire to the battery but all is good. We should all be thankful. We are. We will be able to see her in forty-five minutes.

We are thrilled. We all get on our cell phones and email, contacting everyone we know. Alex's surgery went well! My mom is chaperoning Jessica's all-day field trip to St. Augustine,

Florida. She's been on pins and needles all day. We chose to not tell Jessica about the surgery so my mom has been worrying all day in isolation. My dad calls her immediately. Marc calls his parents. I call my sister. We are so relieved. Now we just have to wait for Alex to wake up.

We wait and wait—much longer than forty-five minutes—and nobody comes to get us. Have they forgotten about us? Is Alex lying in recovery without us? I ask questions of the people in the surgery waiting area but nobody has any information. Dr. Alden comes back. He looks grave.

He says, "Things are not good." I will never forget his face or those words. When they tried to wake Alex, it was difficult. Then they looked at her eyes and her left pupil was blown—dilated in a way indicative of a brain trauma. She had a brain bleed to the left hemisphere of her brain and it isn't good.

Dr. Alden explains they will need to remove a section of her skull to release the pressure and get the blood out. They will leave the skull out so her brain will have room to swell. He says it is very serious, and he cannot anticipate the result. She might not survive. He says he needs to do it immediately. Dr. Alden asks if we have questions. He directs this question to me, clearly anticipating that I will have questions. I always have questions. This time I just say, "No, just go to her. Please help her."

He leaves and we wait and cry. We are panicked. How can this be happening? Things had gone well. What went wrong?

We have to call our family again and give them the bad news. It is tough to even speak through our tears but they have to know. My poor mother has to handle the news while chaperoning Jessica's field trip. I don't know how she is possibly able to hold it together without letting Jessica know.

It is Jessica's birthday.

The Next Forty-Eight Hours

Alex makes it out of surgery after several hours. She is brought back to her room in the ICU and placed into a deep coma. The more inactive we can get her brain the better. The idea is to keep the brain activity down to keep the pressure down. I just cannot be away from her. I have to be in the room with her while the doctors and nurses are getting her situated. The nurses say I can't go in with her but Dr. Alden is here and says that I can and he comes with me. We both stand at the edge of the room, watching Alex and the chaos surrounding her. I stand there feeling Dr. Alden's arm around my shoulder and tears just stream down my face. Marc does not go in the room. He thinks that Alex is about to die. He thinks he will see her brains. He can't get himself to go there. He just paces back and forth in the hallway outside Alex's room. He holds his head in his hands, crying and crying.

As the doctors and nurses get Alex situated in her room, she begins to convulse. She is in pain. How can they let her feel pain? I think the convulsions mean she is about to die. I am in hysterics on the inside but I need to stay calm on the outside or I feel sure they will make me leave. I cannot leave her. It is so awful to watch. Things seem out of control, like what you might see on a TV show. The doctors just keep raising and raising her sedatives until the convulsions stop. She still has a breathing tube so they can get her into a very deep coma.

Before she is brought back to the ICU, doctors place a wire in her brain to measure the pressure. During the chaos around situating her in her room, the wire comes out. The resident has to replace it right there in her hospital room. I feel this could have been avoided. I feel so critical of everyone around her. I want everyone to do better than they are doing but at the same time, I feel sure they are doing the best they can. It is a terrible situation. There are so many doctors and nurses all around her getting things set up as quickly as possible. Her bed is kept on a slant to keep the pressure in her brain as low as possible. The nurses position her head so she is not resting on the side of her head where her skull is missing. That side of her head bulges out. Her scalp is sewn back together; there is a one-inch-wide area where her head is shaved and there are big stitches making a C around the left side of her head. The area protrudes in a sickening way. Before I saw her I had images of her brain hanging out so even though this looks bad, I am slightly relieved by what I see. A cooling blanket keeps her body at a cool temperature and the temperature in the room is set to 55°F, the lowest setting it has. This is to keep her brain as inactive as possible to minimize swelling. There are IVs everywhere, even connected to her central line in her groin.

We are told that if she can survive the next forty-eight hours to four days, her likelihood of making it through this would be significantly increased.

How can we possibly be discussing her likelihood of survival? As the doctors and nurses situate Alex, Dr. Alden continues to stand with me with his arm around my shoulder. He seems so sad.

Tuesday, February 23, 2010 10:28 PM

Things did not go well. Alex had an acute subdural hematoma—a stroke. It was so big that it caused her brain to swell significantly. The neurosurgeon had to remove a palm-sized part of her skull and stitch her back up without it to allow her brain to heal. Her well-being is critical for the next four days and it will be much longer than that before we know the extent of her brain damage, if any. Our hope is that she will be ready to have another surgery in a week or so to replace the part of her skull that was removed and to continue recovery. I know that people will not know what to say and that is fine. I know they all care and are sending good thoughts, love, and prayers. I think that is where we are at and it is appreciated.

—Juli

The ICU doctors act differently around us now, or at least that is how it seems. It feels like nobody makes eye contact with us. Some of the doctors even say things to us as if to prepare us for the worst, such as, "she may not come out of this coma," and "this coma is very serious"—as if we don't already know this. They are so far from helpful. I imagine they are trying to help but really they do the opposite. We are so afraid but also hopeful. She just has to come through this okay. She has made it through the surgery. Now it is our turn to keep her stable. I take this job very seriously. I am impossible to be around.

Alex has to be moved every four hours to keep from developing bedsores. Every time the nurses go to move Alex I stand at the foot of her bed and say, "Be careful, her skull is out on the left side of her head. Don't touch it, don't lean her head that way. Watch her brain pressure!" As if they don't know. Her brain still literally protrudes from her head on the left side. I must remind them a thousand times. I watch Alex's monitor that measures the pressure in her brain. Her neurosurgeon told me that we want to keep that pressure below nineteen while keeping her blood pressure at a safe level. I stare at that brain pressure number so hard as if I can will it to stay low. I am afraid to take my eyes off it. I even limit what I drink so I won't have to leave her to go to the bathroom too often. Alex's brain pressure inevitably goes up slightly when she is moved. I coach the nurses to adjust what they are doing to keep it low. I get into an absolute panic if it nears nineteen. I am quite assertive with my suggestions regarding how Alex should be moved. Her nurses are so patient. I take everything Dr. Alden says as absolute. When he says he wants her body temperature to stay below a certain number, we do everything in our power to keep it there. Her room is like an ice cube. Marc continuously fills reusable ice packs with ice and places them around Alex, against her sides, in her armpits, anywhere we think might help. We all wear long underwear and wrap blankets around us. We keep Alex uncovered and on top of the cooling blanket. Marc admits to using an electric heating pad that Alex had originally taken with her to the hospital during his night shifts. He puts it up under his shirt in an attempt to stay warm.

I wait for Dr. Alden's visits so I can get reassurance from him. He is very careful with how he gives it. He is so attentive to Alex, so concerned. He is the only person I want to speak with. I cannot fathom staying in contact with all the people at home who want—need—updates from me. I send an email to my sister, sisters-in-law, and two closest friends. In the past, when I only sent emails to them, they knew I intended for them to forward the news onto my extended support group. Not this time.

Wednesday, February 24, 2010 1:13 AM

Don't send this email on to anyone. I am sending it to you and a few others to give you a very personal sense of where I am. I don't think my mom should read it at this point.

I will sleep tonight. I have to. I can feel that I am losing control. I know that it is to be expected but I also know I need to do better. I can't seem to stop focusing on the small stuff (a blown IV, for example). It is like I am reading a dissertation and only correcting the grammar. I'm not sure if it is a coping mechanism so I don't have to think about the big stuff or if it is exhaustion—probably a combination. Things have finally gotten somewhat settled. Alex has her brain leads and continuous EEG in place and is in a cold blanket. The nurse is in the room with her monitoring the computer and I will sleep on the parent couch that is also in the room. Marc is in the ICU family lounge and Dad is in a parent sleeping room. Dad has gone the longest without sleep and I cannot bring myself to leave this room so that is how we organized it. The neurosurgeon resident just left. He gave me a sense of what to worry about. Her brain is like someone who has been in a terrible car accident only without the accident and in the OR. The bleed was detected quickly, which is good, but it was not near where they worked to place the DBS so that is somewhat alarming. It was a big bleed and they had to cut away her skull to save her life. If the swelling peaks and begins to go down in the next day or so, then we are a little closer to being out of the woods. We won't know about brain activity until later when they can pull off some of the sedation and begin testing her. The DBS is in place. As you know, that part of the surgery went great and is a positive. Basically, the neurosurgeon described it as this: we have two major things going on here—the issue you went into surgery for, which is certainly not minor and required intubation before, and now this. They are thankful that the DBS is saved. I am so sick to my stomach. Since 3:15 today, I have felt like I am just going to completely break down. I came to see Alex first as soon as she came up to the pediatric ICU from the OR before she was settled or cleaned up and it was awful watching everything, but at the same time I couldn't take my eyes off her. The neurosurgeon (Dr. Alden) came in and just held me. That is when I lost it. In his thirty-two years as a neurosurgeon, he has never experienced anything like this. What is going on????

—Juli

I am living for contact with Dr. Alden and my family is living for contact from me. My emails stop after Alex's surgery, other than the ones I write to a few people. I can't write. I don't know what to say—and that's not minor; I always know what to say. My family is completely isolated. I don't want to have anything to do with anyone but the unit we have become in the hospital: Alex, Marc, my dad, and me. I even have difficulty calling Jessica—I don't know what to say. Marc doesn't contact anyone either; he is too upset. My father calls my mother but she can't call anyone because she is with Jessica. My sister, who lives in Maryland, flies to my mother and Jessica in Orlando. My mother has to take in all this news without any form of outlet, as she has to maintain the safe zone we have created for Jessica. My sister knows my mom needs someone with her. She takes her daughter with her who, like Jessica, is kept unaware of the situation.

Wednesday, February 24, 2010 1:02 PM

I am doing okay again; I have complete hope. Here is the thing. They are now telling me that it is likely she will live. So that is the main thing. As long as we have her, whatever brain damage she has will just be part of our Alex and that is fine.

—*Juli*

Right after hearing the news of Alex's stroke, Sherri, one of Marc's sisters, gets on a plane without asking us and without telling us she is coming. I am so mad at her when I find out she is on her way. Deep down I know it is the right thing to do, but I have so little control over anything that just changing the dynamic of who is at the hospital with Alex puts me over the edge.

12

Family Comes for Support

Sherri comes because she needs to be here. Marc needs her here. We all do, really. We are just sort of surviving in the ICU, we never leave. Different charities and restaurants provide dinners for families of children in the hospital on certain nights. The leftovers are kept in the family kitchen. A bakery brings bagels a few times per week. We eat whatever we can find in the kitchen. When that runs out we eat crackers and cans of soup we find in the kitchen. There are times when there is just nothing around. We don't really have other options as nobody we know lives within hours of this hospital. There is a cafeteria elsewhere in the hospital but we are in no condition to leave the ICU. We just can't leave Alex. We are managing. Sherri organizes dinners to be provided by our family and friends. She finds restaurants that deliver and sets up an online calendar for the family to sign up to be responsible for ordering dinners to be delivered to us on different nights. We don't care what we eat but this is one less thing to deal with. Sherri anticipates needs we don't even know we have. She also provides information to the family. The family needs to have someone who will keep them in the loop; they are struggling too.

Thursday, February 25, 2010 12:22 PM

Alex has a stage-one bedsore; therefore, they are moving her position every two hours instead of every four hours. She also sounds hoarse so they are monitoring to make sure pneumonia doesn't come back. It goes up and down quickly. . . . She was stable and all good until they moved her for circulation. At that time the brain pressure reading went to 18/19 and oxygen levels went down. Marc went quiet and his eyes watered as nurses reacted quickly. Fortunately they were able to stabilize her again. Brain pressure level now 13 of 18 . . . seems 13 is our new norm. They are not concerned and say it was normal for vitals to react as she is moved. They have scheduled her for a CT scan Saturday morning prior to waking her.

Will keep you updated throughout the day via email.

—Sherri

Dr. Alden has to go to California to give a lecture. He is also going to see his new grandson. He cuts his trip short to get back to Alex. He is our glue. He checks in with us on my email and cell phone regularly while he is gone. How amazing is it that he calls us rather than only the ICU? That direct contact is so helpful and so unexpected from a neurosurgeon. I wonder if he even realizes it. I live for that contact so he can tell us everything is okay. He won't say that but he does say that he is cautiously optimistic. He uses that phrase often during this period in Alex's journey.

Thursday, February 25, 2010 6:17 PM

Alex will go for MRI Saturday morning not a CT. Dr. Alden will review MRI on computer in California before he flies back to ensure it looks good to take her out of sedation. He changed his flight to come back Saturday instead of Sunday for Alex.

Her right shoulder is dislocated, probably from moving her around. The doctor says not to try to put it back together while vitals still calm.

They must continue to move her every two hours . . . .

—Sherri

Sending Alex off to have an MRI is traumatic for me. I have been glued to her bedside since she came back from surgery, watching every move the doctors and nurses make, making sure that nothing threatens to raise her brain pressure. I take this job very seriously. One of the nurses tries to keep me away from Alex. I am fairly rude to her in my persistence that she be more careful with the left side of Alex's head. I'm sure I sound on the verge of insanity. She tells me I cannot stay with Alex 100 percent of the time. I can't handle this nurse; after she tries to keep me from my daughter, it feels like my blood boils every time she comes near. I speak with the head doctor for the entire ICU. I have that nurse barred from entering Alex's room. I become extremely assertive in my efforts to protect Alex. Nothing embarrasses me or causes me to relax on my watch. This is another turning point for me, different from when I felt myself shift and back Alex completely during the meeting in New England. In the ICU, I become more single-minded. I don't worry about repercussions for my actions—I just act. If I feel that Alex needs something, I make sure she gets it, regardless of what I have to do. If I feel I need something to be able to protect Alex better, I make sure I get that too. I am sure that some nurses just cringe when they are assigned to work with us; we are not easy on them. It isn't intentional but it isn't anything we worry about either. Marc and I even keep a respiratory therapist from entering Alex's room to check on her breathing tube because the therapist is wearing a mask due to a cold. She says that because she is wearing a mask, she is fine, but we say she is an unnecessary risk. We make her find a replacement. She is not happy but that isn't our problem. Alex is our number one priority. Alex is our only priority. Now Alex will be transported from her room to a different floor of the hospital to get an MRI—without me. The doctors won't let me go with her. Who is going to watch out for her? It is just too much to take. They disconnect her breathing machine and connect a temporary one. I must tell them to be careful about thirty times before they get her out the door. I can't even express the relief I feel when she returns seemingly no worse for the wear. Now we have to wait for the results. They will tell us if Alex has brain damage from the brain bleed. She just has to be okay.

Best-Case Scenario

I think her doctor is waiting as impatiently as I am. He calls me from the airport in California as soon as he sees the results. He is about to board the plane so he has almost no time to look at the results. He says they represent the best-case scenario with what has happened. She is going to be okay!

Sunday, February 28, 2010 11:13 AM

All vitals stable. Same status as last night: Dr. Alden returned from California and visited Alex this morning. He said that MRI results were better than he expected. Alex is stable with brain pressure lowered to ten. They are keeping her sedated today to give her brain one more day to heal and reduce swelling. They will begin extricating her tomorrow morning; it will be a two-day process. As they wake her, there is a strong possibility that the spasms will come back and they are still researching what medication or combined medication they will use to help control the spasms until they are able to turn on the DBS. Hopefully the DBS will work for her. The earliest they will schedule surgery to reconnect her skull is Friday 3/5, and if not Friday, it will likely be after the weekend on Tuesday 3/9.

—Sherri

We are so relieved that she is stabilizing. They keep her in the coma to give her some extra time to heal and that is okay. We are actually afraid to take her out of the coma because of the spasms. Every time we have rounds, we ask the doctors what medications they plan to use if Alex starts spasming. It is especially worrisome because half of her skull is gone. What if she bangs her head? We don't feel like we get a good answer regarding a plan for the spasms. That isn't the only thing that is disconcerting.

We are so excited about the results of her MRI, as is Dr. Alden. Her neurologist does not share the same excitement. Why isn't she excited? This is such great news. Alex's brain is going to be fine! Throughout this process we always talk about how, though it was difficult that Alex had physical limitations, it was with her academics that she had always shone. She was smart, thoughtful, and just deep. We still have that.

Why is the neurologist trying to worry us? She says, "Alex may never be able to speak again. You must be prepared for her to be unable to reason." What is she talking about? She sure is a pessimist. It isn't helpful.

Actually, her reaction is based on information we don't have. There is more to the MRI than Dr. Alden was able to view from the airport in California. Once he reviews the entire set of results from the MRI, he is less optimistic as well. We go from the best-case scenario to the worst-case scenario on March 1, 2010.

Monday, March 1, 2010 1:54 PM

This is my last email from Alex's hospital and probably the hardest to write. Dr. Alden has reviewed the full files of the MRI and has now confirmed some brain damage in the left frontal area that controls speech and other things. No one can say how much damage or how much it will affect Alex until she fully awakens and all the meds are out of her system. Therefore, they are unlikely to have any more information until next week.

I spent the morning with Marc; now I am at the airport to fly home. David (our stepbrother) will be with Marc and Juli from Tuesday to Wednesday and

Valerie (our sister) will be with them Thursday for the weekend.

My heart goes out to them,

—*Sherri*

Worst-Case Scenario

I spend the entire day crying. I haven't really completely broken down and cried since the start of all this. I am always too busy taking care of Alex, being strong for Marc, focusing on the positive. Today everything negative just hits me. I can't stop crying. I don't even sit by Alex's side; I can only grieve. I lie on the vinyl couch in Alex's room. Marc holds me and lets me cry. At some point you just have to let it out. How did it come to this? What will happen next? What have we done to my little girl? Alex is one of my best friends. She has a way of connecting to the world that is just like the way I do. We spent so much time together through her illness. Now the Alex I know and love might be gone. What will I do without her? I cannot stop these thoughts from going through my head. I cannot stop from crying.

When the day is over, so is my crying. I will not let this be the worst-case scenario. She will just have to be okay. I will not believe otherwise. I begin looking for the signs to reassure me.

Code Brown

It is taking a very long time to get Alex off sedation. It is March 4 and she is starting to move her left hand and foot. Her eyes are beginning to open but they are rolled back in her head. She develops a fever that cannot be explained. We check her spinal fluid through the port she still has. Her fluid is fine but the fever is unexplained so she is put on antibiotics.

Alex develops something referred to as C. diff. It can occur when someone takes antibiotics and those antibiotics wipe out important bacteria in one's system. What is important to know about C. diff is that it is very contagious and it causes massive diarrhea; I mean diarrhea like you've never seen before. And the smell—well, it certainly has a distinct smell . . . .

Marc's brother, David, is with us. We really need his help. Alex's left arm sort of flails up toward her head frequently. There is some concern that she might dislodge her breathing tube. We don't want to tie her arms down because we don't want to agitate her or cause any trauma to her, such as more dislocated joints, so Marc, my dad, David, and I set up a twenty-four-hour watch with Alex so that someone is with her—hands on—around the clock to gently guide her arm away from her head whenever it flings up.

I am sitting by her bed with my hands ready to protect her when I hear a sound like water pouring. I look beside me and a brown puddle is forming on the floor next to the bed. "Marc, get a nurse, now! Poop is pouring everywhere!" It is just everywhere. David hits the call button and Marc runs out of the room to get a nurse. Unfortunately it is change of shift, which is a difficult time to get a nurse. The nurses at the end of their shifts need time to meet with the nurses at the beginning of their shifts to update them on their patients. It is a very busy time. The nurse peeks in, takes one look at the situation, and runs for reinforcements. That she is able to get reinforcements at change of shift provides some indication of the mess that Alex is creating.

It takes five nurses to take care of the mess! It is actually pretty funny. They all put on gowns and gloves and get to work at cleaning up Alex who is continuing to gush liquid poop everywhere.

I get out of the way and take my usual position at the end of the bed, reminding the nurses to be careful of Alex's head and her breathing tube. Marc puts on a gown and gloves. But then he just stands in the corner of the room with his hands up in the air like he is about to go in for surgery, just staring at the scene before him. It is like he is in a trance, maybe shock. It sure is a lot of poop.

Alex's bed is in a V shape; her head and feet are slightly elevated. What this results in is a perfect funnel for the flowing poop. We use washcloths to clean her up. We change the sheets repeatedly. I have to leave my post to look for sheets in other empty rooms, as there is no one else available to do so. We use up every sheet and washcloth in the ICU. Each time Alex is cleaned up, her stomach gurgles, and that is followed by the distinct sound of pouring poop. Somehow, it always ends up on the floor no matter how many diapers we layer on her to try to keep it contained. Everything is a mess. It is disgusting beyond words.

Now whenever the nurses see Marc, they hold their hands up in the air like Marc did when he put on the gloves and stood in the corner of the room during the first diarrhea episode. It makes us laugh. It is the only thing that makes us laugh. We also learn a bit more about how things are communicated in the ICU. We hear announcements at various times that something is a code yellow or code blue. We never knew what they meant. After our experience with C. diff we know one code for sure: code brown. We hear it often over the next few days.

13

Holding On to Hope

By the time my sister-in-law Valerie arrives, it is getting more and more difficult to hold on to hope. Every time a doctor or nurse comes in they go through the same routine: "Alex, can you move your fingers?" "Alex, blink if you understand." "Alex, can you squeeze my hand?" Every time there is the same response: nothing.

When the doctors and nurses leave, I go through the same routine. She will surely respond to me. I'm her mother. And yet, nothing.

I try to convince myself she is responding but when I am honest with myself, I know she isn't. I can't take it anymore. I stop watching when the nurses and doctors go through the routine; I turn away. I stop doing it myself. I can't take the constant reminder that my daughter might not be in there after all. Marc calls her "sleeping beauty." He feels she will never wake up, that there is nothing inside. He just watches this beautiful, pale, sleeping child with the sounds of beeping and the breathing machine in the background.

My life with Alex consists of watching monitors, monitoring anyone who comes near Alex, and staying by her side. Marc, my dad, and the nurses try to get me to leave the room to take a break but I just can't. Valerie is the first person who gets me to leave. She was an accountant and has recently started teaching high school math. Numbers hold the same value to her as they do to me. They are almost calming. I am always calculating things mentally while others use computers or calculators. I try to beat them to the solution. Now I find, with my life in the ICU, that I am memorizing dosages of all that is dripping into various parts of Alex's body from the four poles holding bags with fluids and vials with medication surrounding her bed. I memorize Alex's high numbers and low numbers from data displayed on her monitor twenty-four hours per day. I keep track of everything and check the nurses and doctors to make sure they are in agreement. If they are not, I know they are wrong and I am correct and I question them. I know Valerie will keep track of all the numbers on the monitors as well. I know she will be as diligent as I am. I am sure our diligence will be what saves Alex. We have to do what we can to keep her numbers as perfect as possible while she is healing.

Valerie is only able to stay a few days due to her teaching schedule. It is her first year teaching and it is difficult to get away. She sits in Alex's room through the night, watching monitors and grading geometry tests. She behaves so much like me that Dr. Alden takes her to be my sister rather than my sister-in-law. While she is here, I go to the parents' sleeping room and sleep for a few hours. It makes me tense to leave the room, but I know it is necessary. I am so drained.

As Alex continues to come off the medication, we focus on the EEG monitoring her brain activity to ensure she is not having seizures. I find it difficult to stand by while the leads are reconnected every day. They have to be connected to areas where

Alex has no skull. That concept is so scary to me. The moment the technician enters the room, I am on my feet, hovering, looking over her shoulder. The space around the EEG monitor is cramped but I still squeeze myself in next to the technician. "Be careful with the left side of Alex's head, she doesn't have a skull there."

"I know."

"Do you have to reconnect the leads in that area? You're making me nervous."

"They all have to be connected. See the lights on the monitor? They indicate that those leads are not good."

"Okay, just be careful." I stand within six inches of the technician the entire time she works on Alex, reminding her over and over again to be careful of Alex's head. Do these people have to put up with this sort of treatment from the families of all their patients? I can't even imagine it, but that isn't my problem. I only care about Alex. Alex's theme song from New England keeps coming into my head—Alex can lean on me; I will be there to carry her on. This is my single purpose.

The EEG connects to a computer in the room that shows the activity in Alex's brain. The right side has plenty of activity. The left side has none. While I am not exactly sure what that means, I can just feel hope slipping away. The left side of the brain controls Alex's language, cognition, and thought. I look at the series of straight lines. Nothing is going on in that part of Alex's brain. Nothing.

What Do We Tell People?

About the time I begin to feel my hope slipping away, I receive a call from Alex's school. Her classmates want to do something to support her. They want to have a fundraiser to help with our expenses. They want to be able to celebrate Alex upon her return home.

I don't know what to say. How can we raise the hopes of these other children? If they hold a fundraiser and then Alex never makes it home, what will we do? What if she comes home but without much brain activity? I just can't let them do it. I don't know how to begin to explain why.

I can't let the school children know that Alex is in a coma, that she has brain damage. Her own sister doesn't even know. The teachers at Alex's and Jessica's schools do a wonderful job of protecting Jessica. My mother continues staying with Jessica. She even begins volunteering at her school. As a retired elementary school teacher, my mom is loved by everyone there. It gives her something else to focus on. She provides intensive reading support to struggling learners, going from one class to another providing her expertise. She also helps provide a line of communication to Jessica's teachers.

The teachers at Alex's school are so understanding. They offer to come up with something else for Alex's classmates to do, something less public but something that will still provide an outlet for her classmates to express their concern. What a relief. I don't know what they plan to do but I feel glad it will not involve some sort of assembly or public announcement. We just can't go there yet, or possibly ever. We really won't know until Alex is off sedation. It takes forever to get her off the medication.

Withdrawal

Some days are easier to handle than others. Even though I no longer ask Alex to respond to me with a finger squeeze or a blink, I still look for hope in everything—a hand movement, a yawn, anything I can grab on to. It feels like I am riding a terrible roller coaster through the twilight zone.

Monday, March 8, 2010 10:00 PM

Hi,

Today was a good day. The doctors are trying to reduce the meds as quickly as they can so that they can get Alex breathing as soon as possible. That won't happen on the current level of sedation. The plan is to reduce the meds each day as long as Alex tolerates it without going into withdrawal. It is a fine line and different for everyone. She seemed more awake today and she used what seemed like much more purposeful hand movements today, and certainly movements that were much larger than the past. She also pooped, which was a really good thing since she hadn't pooped since Wednesday. She requires a fleet enema to poop, which we hope will change. I imagine she hopes so too. Her stomach is still quite distended and the nurses are all sure she will let loose on their shifts.

Alex will need to have a blood transfusion today or tomorrow. I was hoping to be able to donate my blood for that but the process takes five to seven days so it is not possible, as she needs it now. I wish I had seen that one coming. It is what it is.

The goal now is to extubate her and get her breathing on her own over the next two days. The earliest we are talking about replacing her bone flap is a week from Tuesday.

I'll email again tomorrow.

Love,
Juli

Things just won't go smoothly. Alex goes from constant diarrhea to complete constipation. Now she needs a blood transfusion too; a frequent result of being in a coma for an extended period of time. It is taking longer than anticipated to get Alex off the respirator. With all that Alex has been through, I'm not sure why the thought of a blood transfusion scares me so much. I argue against the transfusion during rounds, asking if we can just postpone it for as long as possible. I am given one more day. As it turns out, her numbers go up and we are able to avoid it. One for the Dixon team . . . but the roller-coaster ride continues.

Wednesday, March 10, 2010 10:47 AM

It was a long night. Alex went into withdrawal last night from going off the drugs too quickly. She had diarrhea, a fever that would go away with each dose of meds, the shakes, and high blood pressure. Her heart rate was in the 180s.

Marc, Dad, and I made a great team but it took all of us almost all night to keep her safe. I have never been so tired in all my life.

—Juli

Withdrawal is awful. It means that we are lowering her medication too quickly. We have to slow down her weaning so she can come out of withdrawal—a difficult situation. Alex has already been on the respirator for seventeen days but we can't take her off it until her medication is low enough.

She is finally off the respirator and now I almost wish she could have it back. Her breathing is awful. I keep thinking she will just stop. The respiratory therapists have to keep helping her to breathe on her own with some sort of treatment. She makes the most awful noise when she breathes. We reposition her head and neck to try to get it to stop. Marc snores, although he'll never admit it, and it drives me nuts. I am always getting on his case about it. I'm embarrassed to say that I will even wake him from a sound sleep to get him to stop. I am overly sensitive to snoring. Now my own daughter has the most obnoxious snore I've ever heard. It is from the breathing tube and it goes away after a week or so but at the time we don't know if she will always breathe like this.

Everything is frightening and unbelievably difficult. As Alex continues to come off sedation she seems to get more and more agitated. It seems like maybe her stomach hurts or she feels uncomfortable. She flails her left arm with such force that sometimes we have to resort to restraining it with a strap and putting a big glove on her left hand. Even when we do this, we need to be right with her to keep her from harming herself. We are so tired. We just can't go on like this. We try to problem solve in our state of exhaustion. Even when it is our turn to rest, we lie awake thinking of what could be making Alex so uncomfortable. Marc comes up with an idea. Alex has always had trouble with soy-based products. Marc has the nurses check the ingredients of Alex's feeding tube contents. It is soy based. We had indicated her allergy in her files but it must have been overlooked. We are probably giving Alex an awful stomachache. We can't help but feel guilty we didn't catch this earlier. Doesn't Alex have enough to deal with? We have to fill her with something that hurts her as well? We only guess this as the culprit but it is the best we can come up with without Alex's help. It reminds me of when she was a newborn baby with colic, but this time I can't call my mom and ask her what to do. We are in uncharted territory here. All we know for sure is our exhaustion.

Marc calls his family and asks for more help. Marc's cousin and his wife drop everything and drive in from Chicago when they get the call. Everyone wants to help us; they just don't know what to do and we don't know what to ask for. When we do ask for help, family arrives.

Sunday, March 14, 2010 2:54 PM

I understand everyone is anxiously awaiting updates; however, there is little news to report. It's great that she was extubated last week and breathing on her own. They are trying to keep her stable to prepare her for the next surgery—tentatively scheduled for Tuesday morning. She remains on a lot of medication so we're unable to assess any cognitive abilities at this time.

Marc, Juli, and Harvey (Juli's dad) have been very tired since they take shifts watching her twenty-four hours/day. Cousin Bruce and his wife Joanne drove two hours from Chicago and stayed with them to help out Friday night. On Saturday, Mom flew to Wisconsin to be with them. Mom will likely stay until Wednesday. If all goes as planned, Jessica may go on Thursday with Joy (Juli's mom) to see her sister.

I will keep you posted as I find out more information.

—Sherri

Alex is breathing on her own but still not responding. Marc and I begin to panic again. Is this how she will stay? Is our Alex just going to lie there with her only action flailing her left arm when awake, needing constant surveillance or to be tied down? What will we do?

14

Saying Goodbye

I have to know what to expect. Dr. Alden comes to see Alex and I ask him outright. I hold my hands apart and say, "When Alex came here, she was a mess physically, but cognitively she was way out here." I indicate one of my outstretched hands. "Now, still somewhat sedated, she is here." I indicate my other outstretched hand. "Where is she going to end up? Will she be closer to my first hand or my second hand?"

The doctor holds his hand quite close to my second hand—the one representing her sedated state—but not all the way there and says, "She will probably be somewhere over here."

"Thank you for telling me." I hear him but I am not ready to absorb what he says. After he leaves, I just climb into Alex's bed beside her and hold her. I cry and cry. I silently say good-bye to the Alex I knew. Marc stands next to the bed with my father next to him. Marc cries and cries as well. We are beyond sad. It feels like an impromptu memorial service.

My good friend and colleague, Lisa, arrives at the hospital in the midst of this vigil, walking into a dimly lit room to witness me curled up around Alex in her hospital bed with my face nestled in the crook of her neck and Marc and my dad somberly looking on. She happens to be in town giving a talk nearby. She comes at just the right time. As a special education professor, she is familiar with issues related with children who have profound disabilities. Lisa suggests that Marc and I go with her to the family waiting room in the ICU to speak about what is going on in our heads. This is the first time we voice our fears. Lisa is a wealth of information at just the right time.

We discuss the possibility that Alex might not ever be well enough to come home. We discuss how we might need to change our home to accommodate her new medical needs if she is able to come home. We discuss the types of nursing support for situations like this. No topic is off-limits. Fortunately Marc and I are of like mind with respect to Alex's care. These sorts of things can rip a family apart. We are determined to keep from being a statistic.

After we voice our fears, we put them to the side, as if we are able to let them go because we let them out. When we come back to the room, we are in a better state of mind. Supporting Alex remains difficult but the entire atmosphere in Alex's room begins to change.

A New Kind of Womb

I'm not exactly sure how this starts but I begin treating Alex as though she is in my womb. I find a CD player and play classical music and Enya in the room around the clock. I read to Alex whenever she is awake. I ask others to read to her too. I feel as though Alex becomes more calm when I read to her or touch her. I touch her as much as I can. I rub her arm, cheek, hand—anything I can get to. I need her to know I am here. I speak to her whenever I am not reading to her; I tell her what is going on around her and who is visiting.

We all do everything we can think of to make her ICU room with all the monitors and IVs as peaceful as possible. It needs to be a place of healing and rebirth. Alex isn't peaceful but her environment is as peaceful as it could be. We even make collages of her numerous cards and pictures and post them all over the walls of her room.

It is finally time for Alex's surgery to replace the part of her skull that was removed. Marc's mom is with us and I feel glad she is there for Marc.

What Will You Dream About?

Every time Alex was put under general anesthesia in the past, I would go with her into the operating room and hold her as she was being put under. Before she went under, the doctor would ask her what she would dream about. During both surgeries since coming to this hospital, Alex has said she will dream about Panda. During the second surgery, it was difficult for her to speak but she still managed to honor the dog she has yet to meet. She also got upset; going under anesthesia frightened her. This time neither response occurs.

Alex is not responsive. She does not speak or show fear. She just lies there. It is heartbreaking. She can't say what she will dream about. I really don't know if she has dreams or knows what a dream is anymore. I don't know if she has fears anymore. I don't know Alex anymore.

My little girl is going back for more surgery and I can't discuss it with her. I can tell her about it but it has been what seems like years since I could discuss anything with her. As I stand next to her operating table in the sterile operating room, my eyes meet Dr. Alden's. I'm sure he knows what I am thinking. It is March 16. Alex hasn't spoken since February 23.

I compose myself as I walk back to meet the others in the surgery waiting area. I have to stay strong for Marc and his mom. I am fairly certain the tension is making me short-tempered with them. It is affecting all of us. When I arrive in the waiting area, I see Marc at a computer terminal. He is googling " brain injury." What he finds is horrifying. We can expect Alex to stay nonresponsive forever. I am not ready to read this. I leave him to continue his search on his own. I can't be a part of it.

Thursday, March 18, 2010 10:47 AM

> Sorry. I forgot to update everyone late Tuesday. Surgery went well. While she was under anesthesia, they were able to brush knots out and braid Alex's hair. No, they did not need to shave her head for surgery. She is off the sedation medications but still on many other medications. It is a difficult and uncomfortable time for Alex. She does attempt to pull out the various tubes and they do at times need to restrain her. They will test her on swallowing and try to get her off the feeding tube shortly. They are still unable to assess any cognitive/recognition abilities at this time.
>
> *—Sherri*

Alex came to this hospital with long hair. It formed ringlet-like curls down to the middle of her back. During her first brain surgery, a strip of hair was shaved down the top of her head and around the left side of her skull. The rest of her hair was left long. During the time she was in a coma, nothing had been done to her hair. It was never even washed after surgery so it still has bits of dried blood in it. She is developing what is quickly approaching dreadlocks. During surgery to replace her skull, the nurses were kind to spend time combing out and braiding her hair while she was under anesthesia. They were able to get to all of her hair other than the part she was resting on. Half of her hair is braided. The rest is still matted. The center of her head is bald with big stitches going down the middle. She is quite a sight. And she is so thin. She was slim when we brought her here. She hadn't eaten for quite some time before she got the feeding tube and then she was on a feeding tube for weeks and weeks. She doesn't look like she did when we brought her here. Jessica is finally coming to the hospital. What will she think when she sees Alex?

15

Jessica

Jessica was born a big baby—eight pounds, seven ounces—but has been tiny ever since. She makes up for it with her vocabulary. She remembers everything and processes it like someone well beyond her years. Her thought process is unusual. When she was younger, we didn't realize she was as academically advanced as she is. We didn't understand the way she made sense of things. As she got older, her intelligence began to shine. She is outstanding in every academic subject while simultaneously lacking common sense—a ten-year-old absent-minded professor. I think she comes across absent-minded because she is always thinking about something else.

She has OCD, but not in the way people commonly think about it. She doesn't straighten everything out; she doesn't turn the light switch on and off over and over. It is more like her brain never shuts off. When she worries about something, she can't stop thinking about it. Often her worries are unreasonable but she can't stop playing them out over and over again in her mind. She is often up for hours in bed waiting for her brain to slow down so she can sleep, and that is with taking melatonin every night. Without it she just doesn't sleep. She has been this way since she was five years old. Jessica's emotions are a great deal more intense and deep than one might expect. Her mental abilities do not match her physique, which makes them even more unexpected.

Jessica is cute. No matter how hard she tries to look like a mature ten year old, she is still cute. Everything about her is tiny except for her eyes. She has to be reminded to eat, which is something I have never understood. She has brown hair and big brown eyes. Her hair and eyes are lighter than Alex's but her skin is darker, a beautiful olive color.

Alex always watched out for Jessica. When kids made fun of Jessica when she was struggling with OCD and wouldn't want to walk on grass or when she went into great detail describing strategies for an outdoor game they might be playing, Alex protected her. Alex included Jessica in all her activities. She didn't seem to have any issues with having her little sister around the way some older siblings often do.

We were all so close. It was difficult for us to be apart for these extended periods and then to come back together in this complicated situation.

Telling Jessica

We are relieved to be getting our family unit together but so worried about sharing the news with Jessica. Will she ever forgive us for keeping this from her for so long? How will she react to Alex? There are so many questions. Marc rents a car so we can meet Jessica and my mom at the airport. We just hold hands silently as we drive to the airport. It is strange to be in a car driving through a town I have lived in for weeks and weeks without ever seeing it. It is difficult for me to leave the hospital even for this short amount of time.

Friday, March 19, 2010 6:22 AM

Good morning,

This might be a long update but I think it is necessary . . . please send it along.

Jessica and my mom arrived early yesterday afternoon. Marc and I were just sick about needing to share such difficult news with Jessica. We felt we needed to be in hugging distance to tell her. Marc and I met them at the airport. This airport is a very comfortable one so we went inside to hang out with Jessica and my mom for a while. We first got caught up with Jessica and how much we missed her. We Skyped with her almost every night but she said that, while Skype provided the ability to hear and see us, she needed the touch. We hugged quite a bit at the airport. Then we told her about Alex.

We told Jessica that Alex had gotten worse so quickly we had to do something to help her live through what was happening to her. She could not go on in the condition she was in. Her muscles were breaking down and no medicine that would allow her to breathe on her own seemed to allow her to sleep. We told her we tried every medicine the doctors here and elsewhere could think of trying. We had nothing left but brain surgery. We told Jessica that during brain surgery Alex's brain started to bleed a lot. We told her it was nobody's fault but just the way Alex's brain reacted to the surgery at that point in time. We made sure she knew it was very rare so that she might be less frightened if she ever needs surgery. Then we told Jessica about the damage the surgery caused to Alex's brain.

We told Jessica that Alex would never be the same as the Alex that Jessica knows but the Alex that Jessica knows and loves would be inside the new Alex. The new Alex might not know how to show Jessica she is there but Jessica needs to believe it in her heart. We told Jessica that Alex may never be able to speak or understand what Jessica says but that Alex will always be able to feel love, as she already shows when she is comforted by our touches or when we read to her. We told Jessica we truly didn't know what Alex would be capable of doing. We all cried over losing the Alex we love so much. We needed to make sure that Jessica could grieve and we believe she began that process.

As Jessica cried and we held her, she began sharing how she would take the role of the big little sister. She said she would teach Alex all she was capable of learning and, no matter what that was, she would always remain Alex's best friend. She asked how long we had known this about Alex and we told her the truth. We also told her who in the family had come to see Alex and help out; we were done with secrets. She asked why we had waited to tell her and we said that we felt that we just HAD to be able to hold her and hug her when we shared the news. Jessica felt that we made the right decision and we all breathed more easily. She then said she was ready to see Alex.

We had already planned for the child life specialist, Kathy, to meet us at the hospital before going to Alex's room. Kathy met us and went over how the hospital was set up and where Jessica could go if she wanted to get away from Alex's room. She showed pictures of what Jessica would see in Alex's room and described the functions of all the equipment. Jessica asked a few questions and then said she'd like to see Alex.

We went into Alex's room and Jessica approached her. She touched Alex's arm and said she loved her. Alex tracked Jessica with her eyes immediately. Jessica looked at Alex's head and then seemed to get a bit shaky. Alex's head is partly shaved (a one-inch strip that curves from the middle of her forehead around to a bit past the back of her left ear) and the incision is clearly visible. Kathy asked if Jessica would like to leave for a while and Jessica said yes. Kathy and I took Jessica upstairs to a library and Kathy checked out a laptop for her to use during her stay and showed her a schedule of the many activities available to her. This hospital is just amazing. Eventually we made our way back down to the room and Jessica was fine there, playing on the computer and spending short periods of time at Alex's bedside or sitting on the edge of Alex's bed.

As for Alex, she did something yesterday that made my heart sing. She smiled for Jessica! I'm sure of it. Then Marc was whispering silly things to her using a silly tone of voice and she smiled. My dad saw it and was sure she smiled but Marc wasn't sure. Later, I was hugging her and she grabbed a fistful of my hair and I was silly about it and she smiled again, twice! So we are fairly sure she smiles appropriately at funny actions and/or tones of voice. Marc's shift ended at four a.m. and I took over this morning. During the transition, Marc said that he was talking to her about farting and she smiled again. Could she understand the word fart? I'm not sure I will write that particular word in our book of accomplishments but could she have understood a word? We really don't know but I will take it for now. Alex finds ways to help us to feel hopeful when we get too tired and worried. She is so amazing even during the worst struggle imaginable.

Alex continues to be weaned off the sedatives. She will likely stay in the ICU until she is weaned over the next week. We will then transition from the ICU to in-hospital rehab. I am not sure how long we will be in the hospital for that but at some point we will transfer from the hospital to either a Florida hospital or rehab facility. We will begin researching that once we begin rehab here and the doctors have some idea of our starting point.

At this point, we know Alex likes to be physically comforted by us. She grabs Marc and me with her left arm, which is VERY strong, and pulls us to her, then she puts her arm around us and squeezes. We know Alex enjoys to be read to; she calms down and tracks us when we read. We also know Alex can smile, and maybe understand the word fart. This is the beginning of a very long road for Alex and our entire family but I finally feel like the road has turned in the right direction. I know it won't take us back to where we were but I also believe we will be able to somehow handle wherever we end up at this point.

I am so appreciative of all the support, prayers, and kind thoughts you have all sent (not to mention the food). Please know that I don't always have the time or energy to show it but please know I love you all. Alex's journey will certainly take a village of support and I am so thankful you are part of our village.

Love,
Juli

Jessica handles the news about Alex and seeing Alex beautifully. I can't even begin to express the pride I feel in my daughter as she so gracefully takes on the role of big sister. She has so much to take in today. She cries quite a bit. She also needs lots of hugs. What probably helps her most is her ability to talk things through. Jessica's unique way of seeing life helps tremendously. She is among one of the deepest, most thoughtful children I have ever come to know. I suppose I'm biased but I'm okay with that too.

It has been weeks with no response from Alex, with no indication that she knows anything of her surroundings. Her sister—her best friend—walks into the room and Alex smiles. It isn't a big smile—one part of half of her mouth curves up—but over the next few days that smile grows until there is no doubt she knows us and has some level of understanding of what is going on around her. The power of family and love and acceptance is awe-inspiring.

THE LITTLE BIG SISTER (BY JESSICA DIXON)

I am talking to Mom on the computer, telling her how much I miss her and need her. She tells me I don't have to miss her anymore. I am going to fly up to see them soon. These words occupy my every thought and every word that I say. I will be able to hug Mom and Dad. I will see my grandfather and be with my sister again. I imagine every little detail of my arrival in my head. I am convinced it will be perfect. Maybe even better than what I imagine.

Every person in my fourth grade class writes Alex a "get–well" card and my favorite one is mine. The other students write one sentence and draw a small picture. I write what most adults call a passage and what most fourth graders call a book. I draw a sweet, meaningful picture of us hugging with a bunch of balloons around us symbolizing a welcome home party. She understands me and I understand her. I will be away from the loneliness and into her arms as the downward spiral of the last few years stops.

My grandma and I pack everything we need. Grandma and I are better now that the cracks in my heart are sealed. We drive to the airport and board our first plane. I look out the window and can't stop talking about how amazing every-thing will be when I get there. I am so absorbed in picturing our joyful reunion that I don't need to open a book or do anything else for the entire three hours on the first plane and the entire two hours on the second plane. I am completely content imagining Alex and me on a bike ride going fast or Alex and me swimming in the pool playing Marco Polo rac-ing away from the searcher. She will stop looking sad and I can become the carefree little sister again.

When we get off the plane Grandma is slightly quiet. Maybe she is thinking about Grandpa. She really misses him. We get ice cream because we are early and head down the moving stairs. After waiting in a chair for twenty minutes I actually get to see my parents come through the automatic doors. It is a sight I will never forget. They look so happy to see me but there is something else in their eyes too.

They sit down and tell me what happened to Alex. Alex isn't responding. Even though Alex is older she is like a baby. In a way I am the big sister, but I am the younger one as well. I tell Mom and Dad the most intelligent thing I've ever said. I tell them I will be the best big little sister ever. In that moment I can visibly see Mom and Dad relax. They were expecting me to break again. They didn't know how much I would hurt. What I say reassures them that I will fight for Alex as much as they will. I am finally part of the fight for Alex even though this time we are fighting the confines of her brain.

We get in the car and drive to the hospital. I talk to Mom and Dad about our plans for the family's new life. They are even talking about moving up here so Alex can become one of the hospital's permanent residents. I don't want to move but I will for Alex.

I take the elevator up to the ICU wing. I walk into the hallway with my parents and a lady appears. She is there to help me. They are all going in with me to meet my "baby sister." When I walk in I think I am prepared for everything. I'm not. I see Alex and she looks the same except for a monster scar running from the front of her head all the way to the back. She has a feeding tube in her nose. I can't stand to look at her scar. It is almost like that scar took Alex away from me. I notice something. Alex is smiling with half of her mouth because the other half is paralyzed. Everyone looks excited. It turns out that this is the first reaction they've gotten from Alex since the coma. Alex, somewhere deep inside of her, knows me. That means more to me than any words that could be said. Good thing too, because Alex can't say any words. I never thought I could be so moved by a simple smile. Well, maybe that smile wasn't so simple.

I talk to Alex like she understands me, but then I leave the room. The sight of her scar makes me upset. I am so upset I have to leave. The lady gives me a tour of the hospital and the stuff I can do there. The hospital is new and shiny. If Alex has to spend her life in a hospital, the best place for her would be here. Soon the afternoon starts to fade and I have to leave the hospital. I am going to stay at the Ronald McDonald House. Dad drives my grandparents and me there. It is a cozy place. I have a room to stay in while I am here. Dad leaves. I have to sleep on the bed next to my grandparents, who both snore really badly. Despite the insane snoring I fall asleep.

During the week, I am here Alex says her first word and passes her swallow test. It is an improvement but my life will never fit my vision. Alex used to be smart and active. Alex now can't say anything other than "noooooooo" and she can't even sit up. I have reached a habit of assuming things people don't tell me. I assumed Alex would get completely better and she is worse than ever now. I assumed the pain clinic would work but it didn't. I guess it is a side effect of when people don't tell me the facts. The assumptions make me happy until I find the truth and then I suffer a letdown. You would think that I would be used to letdowns by now. I often throw myself into a book. Pretending I am the main character momentarily takes my mind off of reality. The sad thing is when I have to close my book I am back into the life of Jessica, the girl with a brain-dead sister.

. . . .

PART III: RECOVERY

16

Bringing Alex Back

We are ready to begin the long process of bringing Alex back to us. She finds ways to communicate with us. It is clear her head is uncomfortable but we feel it bothers her in areas in addition to where she had surgery. We take a closer look and find her hair has become so knotty it is literally being pulled from her scalp. This we can fix.

My mom and I climb in Alex's bed and give her a haircut. We just grab handfuls of hair and snip it off wherever it seems to be pulling from her scalp. I can't say it is a pretty haircut, but considering that she already has a shaved strip down the middle of her head, it isn't a big deal. It makes her so much more comfortable.

The next step is getting her out of bed. She has been lying down for so long she is literally unable to sit up. She cannot maintain the position; her blood pressure drops too drastically. She also doesn't have the strength to hold up her head.

We slide her out of bed onto a chair designed to begin flat and then slowly tilt her up. We strap her in and begin to tilt her up. Each time we try, she slides down in the chair and we need to begin the process all over again. She is difficult to manage. I can't imagine what it would be like with an adult. Alex is only slightly more than eighty pounds. She is about five feet tall—tall enough to reasonably weigh a hundred pounds. How would we have gotten her out of bed if she were within her normal weight range? She is like an unruly sack of potatoes. Just sliding her over to the tilting chair is a huge ordeal. We slide her across a Teflon platform to get her onto the chair that is more like a stretcher. We strap her to the chair in every way we can think and then we begin tilting. As soon as she begins to tilt, she begins to slide. Isn't this something many patients need to do? You would think there would be a better contraption. It seems like we will never get her sitting.

She is still using a feeding tube. To teach her to eat again, she needs to be able to sit up and pass the swallow study; she has to demonstrate that she can swallow food properly so it doesn't go into her lungs. This is the level we are at. First we needed to see if she could breathe on her own; now we need to see if she can swallow on her own. We know so little about Alex's potential. We are basically told that we can count on her being something like a vegetable and we won't accept that. We are going to get her to sit up and swallow. We are not giving up. We finally get her to a sitting position. She cannot hold her head up, so she is in a supported, tilted chair—but she is sitting. She is ready for the study. She hasn't eaten anything in five weeks.

The swallow study is rough. Coaxing Alex to swallow barium in food after not eating for so long and after she has been through so many traumas is next to impossible. It almost *is* impossible. The technicians are ready to give up before I am. I cannot get Alex to cooperate. She seems fussier than normal. I try to think of what I did when she was fussy as a baby. It was so long ago but I remember that I would check her diaper! I check and that is the culprit. I convince the technicians and nurses to wait while I change Alex's diaper while she is sitting in the chair. This was much easier when she was the size of a baby. It is no small accomplishment and it takes much persuading to get all involved to wait. I am Alex's advocate—she cannot advocate for herself—the job is important. I am comfortable asserting myself so people will wait for me to think things through and work things out. I think back on when I began advocating so strongly. It all began when I turned into the Hulk and became ingrained during rounds in the ICU. This story would have ended differently if I hadn't become comfortable in this role.

Saturday, March 20, 2010 7:51 AM

So now that Alex passed her swallow study, we can begin to teach her to eat again. We are to practice twice per day with either pureed food or liquids. Of course, I tried ice cream last night. She did great. It is so strange to have to reteach these things. Her tongue doesn't work well yet so it is difficult to move the food. She also has trouble coordinating when to open her mouth. But she is my daughter so I know that if she will accomplish anything, it will be eating.

Eventually, I put the spoon in her left hand and helped her to guide it to her mouth; with just a little tug on her chin she was able to open her mouth and feed herself. Then she would forget to swallow (remember she is still somewhat sedated), but if we rub her cheek a little she is stimulated to swallow. She did just great for her first attempt. I can't wait to try it again today.

I feel like I am sharing such tiny little things but they truly are monumental, as I'm sure you know.

It is nice to have a place to share them. I'm looking forward to sharing more great things. However, I've been warned that Alex's journey will be more like the frog jumping out of the well with two jumps forward and one jump back. I need to prepare myself for the backward jumps. We might have one today as she will need additional sedation for her MRI. Here's hoping we still get at least one jump forward.

—Juli

P.S. I had to stop typing this for about thirty minutes. Alex just had diarrhea so bad that it went all through and out her diaper and over the side of the bed and poured onto the floor—and I mean poured. It was pretty funny since I don't much like her nurse this shift. . . . It's the little things.

It is so nice to have things to work on with Alex rather than to just sit with her and watch monitors all day long. With her skull back in her head and her breathing tube out, we are also less afraid of her and for her. It was difficult to feel comfortable with her when her brain was pushing out against her scalp and a tube was down her throat breathing for her. Now we climb in bed with her and cuddle her more easily. I am purposeful about having a lot of physical contact with her. When I climb in bed with her, I get under the covers and scoot my body up behind her and wrap my arm over the top of her. My face cuddles in to the back of her neck. She is so thin and vulnerable. I wrap myself around her physically as much as mentally. We do this with babies when we hold them and nurse them. In a sense, I see Alex as a newborn again. She can't do anything for herself. She can't talk. She can't control her movements. She can't even sit on her own. We need to reteach her all that we had taken for granted for so many years. We did a great job the first time. We will do it again.

We put all of our energy into helping Alex recover. We make sure her room is positive. We keep it bright and cheery with the shades up, pictures on the walls, and balloons floating in the corner. We read and speak to her throughout the day and patiently help her to learn to eat again. The MRI is scheduled for March 20 and it will give us an indication if any of our efforts will pay off. Alex will be in the MRI without me, and that makes me feel uncomfortable.

I go from feeling uncomfortable to feeling downright mad. I have grown accustomed to making sense of Alex's cues, responding to her actions. I expect the same behavior from all who work with her. I expect doctors, nurses, and technicians to make sense of her actions as forms of communication. It takes time, patience, and the willingness to be a problem solver. The radiologist that gives her the MRI does not perform to my expectations. This is another example of a doctor not "listening" to Alex. She can't speak up for herself now and I wasn't allowed to go to the MRI with her. She was agitated and moving around. Rather than taking that as a form of communication, the radiologist and technicians just drugged her. If they had stopped to assess the situation, they could have changed her diaper and likely avoided her having to endure yet another breathing tube. Times like this cause me to completely lose my cool. I become so angry and nasty with my remarks that Marc needs to rein me back in. I can handle Alex's condition but not the somewhat minor, unnecessary injustices.

Saturday, March 20, 2010 5:41 PM

Alex just got back from the MRI. She was given a breathing tube during the process, which shouldn't have happened and I am livid about that. She is now extubated and recovering in our room. They gave her morphine because they said she was so agitated, but of course they never checked that she had a diaper full of poop before drugging her to calm her down . . . .

The MRI Alex had on February 27, four days after the brain bleed, presented the worst-case scenario for us. It showed that Alex had possible brain damage throughout the entire left hemisphere of her brain. The MRI today was better than that worst-case scenario. This MRI shows atrophy in part of the occipital lobe and some damage to the area that controls memory, communication, and right-side movement. While we still do not know how this will play out, we now have hope we did not have before for a better recovery. It is likely that her vision will be affected. Dr. Alden says she might not see to the right side from both eyes. We just don't know yet.

So we are cautiously optimistic. We know what looks like less than major damage can have major repercussions but that is still often better than the results of major damage. We also know Alex DOES have brain damage and will not come out of this without some changes. However, what we feel is renewed hope and we wanted to share that feeling with you.

Love,
Juli

It is time to focus on rehab. That means that we need to wean Alex off her remaining sedation. Dr. Alden feels there is about a 40-percent chance that the spasms will return once the medication is completely out of Alex's system and, if that occurs, it would be better if we were still in the ICU. He hopes the damage to the surface of the left hemisphere of Alex's brain is enough to resolve the issue of the overstimulation it communicated, the likely cause of the spasms.

Marc, my mom, and Jessica plan to go home once Alex is off the medication and transfers out of the ICU. Jessica needs to get back to school and Marc needs to get back to work. He has missed six weeks. My dad will stay with Alex and me. I don't know what I would have done without my parents.

Family Life in the ICU

Jessica and my mom have been in Wisconsin for five days. We find ways to spend time with Jessica outside of the hospital. I need to reconnect with her and focus on her rather than on Alex. That is difficult—not because I don't love Jessica, but because Alex's needs are so great and she is so vulnerable. I feel terribly frightened to leave her side.

Jessica and I go outside to find snow on the ground—a big deal for a child who has spent most of her life in Florida. We go to the church grounds across the street from the hospital and stomp a smiley face and heart in the snow. We do it so it can be seen from Alex's room. We know Alex can't see it but we still make it for her. Everything we do, we do for Alex, whether she knows it or not. Nobody minds it this way. It is just how our lives have turned. We make the most of our time together.

Alex begins to interact more. My dad has a funny game he plays with her. It is the same game he played with her twelve years earlier when she was just a little baby. He pulls the blanket over her head and says, "Where's Alex?" Then he pulls it down and says, "Here she is!" He does it over and over again. It brings the smile, beginning to spread to the right side of Alex's mouth and into her eyes every time. Eventually she plays it with him. She sees him and uses her left hand to pull her blanket toward her head on her own. She can't make the movements happen just right yet—she can't seem to coordinate her body to move the way she wants and she can't get the blanket up over her face—but her intent is there. She participates and has a sense of humor. Life gets better every day.

Alex likes to have her grandpa near her. She holds his hand when he sits near her bed and she won't let go for what seems like hours. My father loves it.

We still run shifts so that someone is awake with Alex twenty-four hours per day. Marc and I now begin the night with Jessica at the Ronald McDonald House. In the middle of the night, my dad drives over to the house and picks me up to go back to the hospital to relieve my mom. He brings her back with him, then Marc comes back to the hospital with the car. Jessica sleeps through the exchange. It works. Marc and I get time with Jessica and with each other. We keep the car rental for this purpose while Jessica and my mom are with us. That is the only time I sleep away from the hospital and Alex.

We enter a comfortable rhythm in our crazy world. All of these subtle shifts point to entering the next phase of healing. Alex will begin rehab soon. She needs to be moved from the ICU. The idea seems both wonderful and unnerving.

Monday, March 22, 2010 9:57 AM

Marc, my mom, and Jessica will go home over the weekend so that Marc can return to work on Monday.

He needs to do so to protect his job. If Alex's spasms return, we may need to form a new plan but we will cross that bridge if/when we get to it. That leaves one week with just my dad and me until Marni, my sister, gets here the weekend before April 5. It is much easier now because Alex is not grabbing at her feeding tube or head so violently. It truly took all of our strength to keep her safe when she was doing that. She now seems to know that she cannot pull it out. She just pushes on it to reposition it, making no attempt to pull it out. It must be uncomfortable.

So, saving the best for last, I need to tell you that Alex said a word yesterday! I finally took a daytime nap and slept for three hours, which was amazing seeing as I never get to sleep for longer than that, even at night anymore due to our shifts. Well, while I was sleeping I missed everything. Jessica lost a tooth and Alex said "no" twice in response to questions. It was clearly difficult to get the word out but she did it. Mom said that during her shift this past evening she could tell that Alex was trying to mouth other words. She better have been working on "Mom" as I told her that needed to be her next word since she said "Dada" first as a baby.

Sorry for another long update but there seems to be so much to share these days.

Love,
Juli

Preparing to Part

Marc is in no shape to go home alone with Jessica and I am in no shape to take care of Alex alone in the hospital so far from home. My parents, who have been apart for six weeks, prepare to be apart as long as necessary to support us.

I find it hard to send Marc and Jessica home and I know my dad struggles with saying good-bye to my mom. I can't even fathom what it must be like for Marc to leave. I can barely even get myself to leave Alex's hospital room to go down the hall to take a shower. I rarely wash my hair because it takes ten extra minutes. I couldn't have done it. I am on family medical leave from my job. If that hadn't been possible, I would have had to leave my job and face the consequences later.

Marc and I are good support for each other. Tragic events like this one often tear families apart and they certainly wreak havoc on marriages. We had our struggles, especially when Alex first got sick. We would argue about how tough to be with her, but our fights weren't big ones. Marc and I shared a frank discussion on the topic when Lisa visited and we discussed what life might be like with Alex in this condition. We had acknowledged the statistics regarding families in these sorts of difficult situations; they often end up in divorce. We both agreed we were in it for the long haul but that meant we would not have much time for one another in the short term. We would have to be okay. I guess that's how math types handle these sorts of things. Because we know the stats, we know what to avoid. With that we move on, knowing we have agreed to be there for each other. I cannot even imagine having to deal with marriage issues on top of all our struggles. We are fortunate to be of like mind.

While it feels challenging to have Jessica with us living this strange life between the ICU and the Ronald McDonald House, it is still a life and we once again become a family unit.

Jessica quickly becomes part of the team. She accompanies me to "rounds" when the doctors congregate outside Alex's door to review her status and discuss options. I have long since been an active member of that team. When Jessica arrives she has almost as many questions for the doctors as I do. The doctors keep asking how old she is because her questions are so far beyond what you would expect from a child her age. She asks why it is difficult for Alex to eat and why she needs a swallow study. When she is told that it takes fifty muscles to swallow, the next day at rounds she asks how many of those fifty muscles are involved with smiling and why Alex can smile more with one side of her mouth than the other. She is comfortable conversing with the doctors and interested in learning anything she thinks might be useful in Alex's recovery.

When Do We Start?

It seems like things are moving fast while at the same time so very slowly. It is difficult to explain, but it does provide an important perspective on just how far Alex has to go.

Now that Alex is out of her coma and somewhat responsive, she begins to have visits from therapists. Physical therapists come and move her legs and put her in all sorts of contraptions to help her legs to stay healthy and to try to stretch her right leg. They place soft plastic wraps around her legs and connect them to a motor that fills them with air and then sucks the air out repeatedly to guard against blood clots. She wears big boots with straps to pull her toes up so her Achilles tendons won't get too tight. It seems we are constantly putting things on and taking things off her legs.

Occupational therapists work on her right hand and arm. It is particularly difficult for them because Alex's shoulder was so badly damaged during all the spasms that they can barely move it without it coming out of socket. Speech therapists work on helping Alex to regain the mechanics of eating. It seems to take so much effort just to master when to open her mouth for food. It will take a village to bring Alex back.

Tuesday, March 23, 2010 6:03 AM

Alex continues to work so hard to do the things she used to do. At times she gets frustrated, but mostly when she is uncomfortable and we cannot figure out why. Yesterday evening at rounds Dr. Alden said he had never seen a brain bleed as bad as Alex's and he has also never seen a recovery with such great acceleration in his thirty-two years as a neurosurgeon. It is hard to believe, and yet, it is so Alex. She is trying to talk now. She is very difficult to understand since her right side still looks like she had a stroke but she said, "I want Mama," last night. You can probably imagine how quickly my heart melted.

Dr. Alden asked Alex to move her right arm and she moved her hand a little. He said that was even better than moving her arm at this point. He is hopeful that she might regain some movement on her right side.

Alex started watching TV yesterday, and I mean truly focusing. Jessica climbed up and cuddled with Alex in her bed. It was just like home. Alex has not said "Jessica" yet. Jessica told Alex she knows that "Jessica" is a hard word to say. She said Alex could call her anything she wants and she started listing a very long list of options. It was so cute. Jessica has been so good about not being the center of attention. We work hard to do things with Jessica but the truth is that she is spending quite a bit of time reading in Alex's room.

We stopped the twenty-four-hour watch last night. I slept in Alex's room while she slept. I slept six hours and I don't know what to do with myself! I haven't slept that long in ages.

Take care,
Juli

It is amazing to see measurable changes. If I think about it, I guess the changes are pretty small—like being able to watch TV—but huge in comparison to where Alex was when the doctors asked her to blink her eyes and got no response. It truly seems like rebirthing a child. She goes through stages of movement, communication, reasoning somewhat—as if developing from baby to child but in fast-forward.

We are looking forward to starting rehab in earnest. The issue is that Alex might not be ready to start. She needs to be able to focus long enough and have enough strength to withstand thirty-minute therapy sessions several times per day. She isn't there yet. She can't sit up with someone supporting her for more than a few minutes at a time. She can't sit on her own at all.

If she isn't ready for rehab shortly after returning to the regular floor from the ICU, then we will have to leave. The hospital won't be able to keep us here. Where will we go? We know she needs in-patient rehab, so how can we possibly be sent away? These stresses layer themselves on top of the immediate issues related to Alex's well-being. We don't even know if rehab will be covered by my insurance. Luckily we have two insurance policies. Marc's insurance covers much of what mine will not. Our story would have been much different if not for this—another reminder of how lucky we are. Most families do not have two insurance policies.

Alex is returning to us. We credit her inner strength, her family's support, and the efforts of the village that has formed to support Alex within this hospital.

Wednesday, March 24, 2010 11:21 PM

We continue to see great progress with Alex and she is funnier than ever. It is amazing that she is easier to understand since just this morning. This evening her nurse was doing the nightly evaluation and asked Alex to squeeze her hands and wiggle her toes. Alex cannot wiggle her right toes. When the nurse asked her to, Alex said, "Wiggle, wiggle, wiggle," in place of wiggling her toes. I guess you had to be there, but it was the funniest thing ever, especially since the nurses, rehab therapists, and doctors are constantly so surprised by what Alex can do.

Her reasoning seems to be improving quickly as well. She was able to change the channel on the hospital TV remote. That is such advanced thinking that we are thrilled, even if she did pick the Disney Channel.

She is doing well with getting the spoon of food we give her into her mouth now, but once it is in her mouth she just cries and cries. We think she might have broken a tooth during the spasms before surgery. An in-hospital dentist will see her soon to check. She also has quite a bit of trouble sitting up. I guess that makes sense after being completely bedridden for six and a half weeks. However, while she was sitting on the side of the bed with assistance, she was able to toss a plastic ball, knock over plastic bowling pins, and then count the five pins that remained standing. I'm just glad we are finally working on math.

Today we tried to do something about her hair. It was just too far gone. The matting was so bad that her hair was literally being pulled from her scalp. We had the in-hospital beautician come and cut her hair. When she cut the matted portion away, I was so surprised to find that the back of her head is just bald. I guess all those weeks of being bedridden wore off her hair. I wouldn't say she has the best style now with the stripes that are shaved off, the long pieces on top, the incisions, and the bald spot, but she looks pretty darn cute to us.

Love,
Juli

Alex isn't too happy about the beautician's visit. First, the beautician has to wash Alex's hair while Alex lies down in bed. She uses this sort of miniature blow-up kiddie pool just large enough for Alex's head, a bit of water, and the beautician's hands to fit. There is a dip in one side for Alex's neck. It has a drain in the bottom to let the water out through a tube we stick in a plastic garbage can. It works for the most part but Alex's bed does manage to get pretty wet. It takes Marc, my mom, the beautician, and me to get Alex's hair washed. Alex's head feels sensitive and she doesn't want anyone to touch her hair. She fights us the entire time. The beautician remains positive. I can't say the same for me.

After washing Alex's hair, the beautician basically climbs in Alex's bed to cut it. By the end I wish Dr. Alden had just shaved her entire head during surgery.

With her new haircut, Alex is ready to leave the ICU. The ICU is not a place you want to go, but once there, it is not a place you want to leave. It provides a sense of security because there are always nurses and doctors available to you right outside your door. The regular floor clearly has support but it is different. I feel so afraid to be transferring, even just to the other side of the same hospital floor. It feels similar to the feeling I had when I first brought Alex home from the hospital as an infant. I will need to do more on my own with her.

I remind myself of the reasons we are ready to move: Alex's spasms have not returned, she is more aware, and she is breathing well. We are very close to entering the next phase of her recovery.

17

Moving Out of the ICU

It amazes me how much stuff we have accumulated in a month and a half. So many people have sent Alex care packages. Volunteers at the hospital give her handmade blankets and pillowcases. The balloons sent to her refuse to deflate and I don't have the heart to dispose of them. There are so many that they remind me of the movie *Up*. Rather than pay attention as the stuff accumulates, I just keep shoving stuff in cabinets and corners. We never go home, so everything we are given stays with us. Moving from the ICU to the new room outside of the ICU is almost embarrassing. We have to make several trips with a cart.

The new room has a different view. We had spent well over a month in the ICU in the same room. I had contemplated so much while looking out the window. It seems strange to look out a different window. It also seems strange that Alex lived in the same room for all this time and never even saw out the window.

Thursday, March 25, 2010 11:31 PM

We transferred out of the pediatric ICU to the regular floor today. Today was a steady day with no major improvements. I think I got spoiled with Alex's amazing pace of recovery and so I found today difficult to take. Alex spends much of the day agitated and Dr. Alden says that is common with brain trauma.

There was also good news in addition to Alex's transfer to the regular floor. During PT/OT today, the therapists asked Alex to name each one of us and she did, including Jessica (thank goodness). However, when they showed Alex a sign that said HUG MOM, she just looked at it. They asked her to name the letters and she counted them. She might not be able to read as a result of the damage. I had lulled myself into thinking that all would be back to normal and that was dangerous. However, as I sit next to Alex's bed now, I see a child who is peacefully sleeping with no pain on her face and I feel reassured.

Love,
Juli

We are learning more and more about Alex's condition every day. She can come up with some words. She knows us. She has a sense of humor. She can't read. It is very difficult to keep from focusing on what she can't do. How can she not read? She doesn't even know what letters are. Where does that knowledge go? How do you get it back? It seems so strange to have some parts of Alex but not other parts. Whether we can rebuild the missing parts remains to be seen.

Sometimes I feel that the doctors and therapists feel it is unlikely. I try to ignore those times to the best of my ability. When we are reminded of Alex's limitations, like when she is asked to read "Hug Mom" and she doesn't seem to even understand the words, Marc and I just look at each other. Our looks are filled with a mix of disbelief, dismay, and hope. I think I feel more hopeful than Marc. He is ready to accept Alex the way she is and make the best life possible. I am not satisfied. I want my Alex back. I feel my role beginning to change again. For the past two years I was Alex's medical advocate, fighting for her health and well-being even during those years when my alliance and ways of supporting Alex transitioned. My emerging role: her teacher who requires a different skill set but one of equal importance to her survival.

She needs to stay motivated and proud of every small accomplishment. I need to find a way to maintain her belief in herself while simultaneously instilling a belief that she can do better. I will push her as hard as I need to bring her back. My challenge won't be whether I can push her hard enough; it might just be that I need to be careful not to push her too hard, especially if my own experience of pushing myself is anything to go by.

My parents started me downhill skiing when I was just four. I began figure skating at about eight. By my teens I was quite good at both. However, that wasn't good enough for me. I had to be the best. I pushed myself. I continued to skate through the beginning of college. I would go to the rink early in the morning and practice my axel, a jump where you take off facing forward, spin one and a half revolutions in the air, and land facing backward. I broke my hand during a bad attempt at an axel and had to get a plaster cast. I continued to skate with the cast until I broke that too and I received a fiberglass cast. I was thrilled to discover I could hold my ski pole with the fiberglass cast. I proceeded on a ski trip with my cast. As the ski group learned to jump, I felt excited because I hoped my figure skating background would help me to excel. I tried to pull off a helicopter. That is when you jump, spin a full revolution in the air, and land facing downhill. I tried so hard that I spun one and a quarter revolutions and landed facing perpendicular to the hill (I guess I was still working on my axel in my mind). My body kept rotating and I tore the ligaments in my ankle. Unable to maneuver around the snowy campus, I was sent home from college with casts on both my ankle and my hand. Less than a month later, I performed in a skating show with my hand in a cast and my figure skate taped to my braced ankle. I could not let my skating team down. I never give up and I often push myself harder than was wise. Will I do this with Alex?

Lifting Alex

We are working on getting Alex out of bed and out of her room. Alex only weighs about eighty-three pounds. You would think she would be easy to get out of bed. Not so. Her right side is paralyzed, her right arm sort of hangs out of its socket, she can't hold up her head, and she can't follow a string of basic directions. When we try to maneuver her, it feels like lifting an octopus. However, she is fairly compliant.

There is a lifting contraption above her bed in her hospital room. It consists of a sling-like seat and an electronic lifting mechanism. We strap her in the sling and hook the sling on the lifting mechanism. Once accomplished, we press the UP button on the lifting mechanism to raise her up and move the mechanism along a track until Alex hangs over the tilting wheelchair. All that is left is to lower her into the wheelchair and unhook and remove the sling. That seems easy enough, but in practice it is not so easy.

Every time we try to lift our skinny and weak Alex, she sort of sags through the bottom of the sling. Her butt just slips out. She thinks this is funny. Sometimes we make it farther than others; sometimes we get her all the way lifted up and moved partway to the wheelchair; but at some point her butt always slips through. This sling is clearly not designed for thin children. We are in hysterics laughing. Marc is a professional engineer, my dad has a Ph.D. in science education, and I have a Ph.D. in mathematics education. We know we have the brainpower to do this. As problem solvers, we are determined to rig the contraption to work. The nurses just stand by and let us have at it. We wrap Alex up in the sling in every possible way before we finally give up and lift her with her butt hanging out of the sling about a foot below her body.

We finally get her in the wheelchair. After all that she doesn't like the wheelchair. I thought she would be thrilled to get out of her room. Her brain can't take all the stimuli; the lights, commotion, people, and noise are too much. Just sitting reclined in the tilting wheelchair exhausts her. Apparently even getting her around in a wheelchair successfully will be a long process. We are in it for the long haul. We decide to focus on small accomplishments. We get her out of bed and in the hall for five minutes and she does not enjoy it. We will work to do more next time. People seem to be proud of her progress, so we will be too.

Saturday, March 27, 2010 1:36 PM

I'm so excited to share another terrific update. Dr. Alden was here this morning and after he interacted with Alex he told us this has been the most outstanding eight days of recovery he has ever seen. She even knew who he was. Prior to her surgery, Dr. Alden would always tell Alex she could ask him three questions and she would, every time. Today I asked Alex if she wanted to ask Dr. Alden a question. She looked over to him (indicating that she knows who he is) and tried to ask a question. She was not able to get the question out but she clearly had one. I told her she could wait and ask tomorrow.

Alex is talking more. The speech therapist gave us some strategies to help Alex get to phrases and they are working well. She is holding her head up much better and she is getting around on the bed. She can roll herself onto her side to sleep.

There is some concern regarding the position of her right shoulder (the one with the thousands of dislocations during her spasms). It was taped in place yesterday. She is also unable to pee so she needs to be catheterized every six hours, which is clearly no fun. A pediatric urologist will see her soon to address that issue.

Alex continues to be very affectionate with us and we can't get enough of her. Here's sending you warm Alex hugs to share as well.

Love,
Juli

We focus on the positives but we don't ignore the negatives. They are part of her too. Her shoulder is a mess. You can fit at least three finger widths between where her shoulder is and where her arm starts. It just hangs out of socket. No sling or brace device and no amount of tape seem to be able to hold it in. More pressing at this point is her inability to void her own urine.

Rethinking Daily Living

The urologist examines Alex and runs some tests. He concludes that Alex might never be able to pee again without being catheterized. Well, that isn't exactly how he explains it but the gist is the same. Meanwhile, the nurses have a very difficult time catheterizing her. If she isn't going to be able to pee without being catheterized, then I need to learn to do it and I better do it well. Alex has enough to deal with without having to be put through six failed attempts before success every time she needs to pee.

I ask the urologist to show me how to catheterize her. I figure I should ask the expert. He shows me and I feel much better. If this is going to be our new way of life, then we better get used to it. After the urologist shows me how, I am able to catheterize her successfully the first time every time. I won't let anyone else do it. Alex and I sort of get it down to a routine. She is able to help a little by holding either the wipes or the catheter. It seems bizarre to think she will have to live like this. Every time things seem to approach a sort of normal, we have our boat rocked again.

The dips tend to be balanced by celebrations as Alex continues to heal. It is so rewarding to see her participate in more of her daily living. For so long she even had machines to breath for her. She is beginning to talk now. People often say we should use our strengths to counter our weaknesses. This is never as evident as when we help Alex to find her words.

18

Finding Words

Most of Alex's right side of her brain is intact. That is where rhymes and songs are stored. Imagine—a child who does not remember her own name or the word "Mom" most of the time, she can't read or write or recognize letters, but she *can* sing all the words to a Hannah Montana song. It is bizarre. She is only just beginning to say very short sentences and not often. When she tries to say sentences we have to cue her for several of the words. Then we put on a Hannah Montana CD and she sings all the words. We use what she can do to help her get to what she can't reach. We begin speaking in nursery rhymes. First we need to figure out what she wants to say, then we come up with a rhyme or saying that she already knows. We say the rhyme or saying, leaving out the word she wants to say. She then says the word and feels successful. We use that success to help motivate her to continue trying to talk. For example, if we are having her identify pictures and there is a picture of a star, we might need to say, "Twinkle, twinkle little . . ." and she says, "star."

Alex wants to talk. Talking is her thing. She began talking very early as a toddler—remember when she was interviewed for the video at age five and she said she wanted to be a farmer? At the time, the cameramen could not get over how much she spoke. Well, she wants to speak again and we need to use that motivation while being careful to minimize the frustration. This proves challenging. It works out great when we can figure out what she wants to say. It is not so successful when we can't. We play a strange form of charades whenever we try to communicate.

As her endurance increases, we push her around the hospital in her wheelchair and have her try to name the animals in pictures on the hospital walls. She gets most of them wrong but we don't give up. We won't let her give up either, even when she becomes frustrated. We just keep pointing out pictures and asking her to name them or tell us what they "say."

Probably the funniest part of her speech is how she gets stuck on certain words or phrases. She knows it is wrong but she can't stop saying it. That is part of her brain damage—it involves her inability to "find" words and also a tendency to get "stuck" on other words.

When we get to the pig, we say, "a pig says . . ." and she says, "oink, oink." The funny part is that after she says, "oink, oink" once, she can't seem to stop. She keeps saying it over and over. This becomes a problem when it is time to go back to her room. Our favorite nurse on this floor is overweight. We just love her. We feel so afraid that if we bring Alex back to the room while she is still stuck on saying "oink, oink" the nurse will feel offended. We end up on quite a few unplanned, extended walks around the hospital due to this issue. These are some funny times.

My dad and I are in hysterics during several of our walks around the hospital; people must think we are crazy but I don't care. I strongly believe that humor helps to heal and because of that I try to find reasons to laugh often. It helps that Alex is so funny. She seems to like to laugh as well. I find it strange to see how many gaps she has, but even with her very limited ability to speak she manages to purposefully say such funny things.

Tuesday, March 30, 2010 8:35 PM

We are working on building Alex's endurance to begin rehab. The hope is that she will begin on Monday. In the meantime she is getting short sessions of rehab (PT/OT/speech/eating) daily. She is improving every day. The doctors and therapists are amazed. She is a celebrity at the hospital. People read her report and come in to see her with their own eyes. With that said, Alex still has a long way to go.

She is beginning to talk but she needs quite a bit of help doing so. She loses words and gets stuck on others. For example, if she recognizes a picture of a dog and calls it a dog, then she sees a picture of a pig, she will also call it a dog. But if you say, "Think of 'the three little . . .'" she will say "pigs." It is very interesting. She is beginning to use sentences with some help. Two days ago, we asked her if she had a question for Dr. Alden and she asked, "How can I get my body to work?" Today she asked, "How can I talk?" This is a major accomplishment. She clearly has logic and reasoning and she can talk, so much more should follow. She does not recognize letters or numbers but she does know they are letters and numbers, which is a good start. We are not yet sure she will be able to read but we are hopeful.

She has mastered the mechanics of eating but she is not interested in eating. I think we are still feeding her through her feeding tube at too great a rate, but she has lost so much weight that the nutritionists are apprehensive about lowering her level. I think eating will come—she can even use a straw!

Physically, Alex is regaining strength and control. She can do everything with her left arm, she can hold up her head, and she can sit unassisted for a few seconds at a time. She is in a wheelchair for an hour at a time and she holds her head off the headrest on her own. She can move her right arm slightly with a great deal of effort. She cannot move her right leg yet. We were using a hoist to get her out of the bed and into the wheelchair. This afternoon she began helping to stand on her left leg to get from the bed to the wheelchair and back without the hoist. That opens up much more freedom.

What I am most thrilled about is that Alex's sense of humor is back. She is so funny and is just great to be around. She has been such a trooper through some really awful things. I love every minute I spend with her, which is pretty good for an almost-teenager.

Marc, Jessica, and my mom flew home yesterday. Marc had to get back to work and, while Jessica did great here, it was really time for her to focus on other things as well. My mom will continue to stay at our house to support Jessica. I really do credit Alex's turnaround to Jessica's presence. It was difficult for them to leave. Alex told them she loved them and was very sad. She seems to understand most of what is going on.

When Alex is not in rehab, she sleeps, watches videos, or gets read to. My biggest challenge is finding books that hold her interest but are not too confusing. So far, *Because of Winn Dixie* has been the winner.

So, I think that is about it. We are thrilled with her speed of recovery as is everyone here, and at the same time we are impatient for her to recover more.

Love,
Juli

It feels awful to send Jessica, Marc, and my mom home. It is just my dad and I left with Alex so far from home. We don't know when we will see them again. We can't count on how Alex will progress from one day to the next. She runs into some obstacles.

Another Setback

Alex still takes the medication for her RSD pain. In addition to her spasms stopping, her RSD pain is gone. I feel so relieved to see Alex without pain on her face. A child in pain is just the worst, especially when you are so helpless in giving them respite. We begin weaning Alex off the medication intended to reduce her pain shortly after Marc, Jessica, and my mom leave. She no longer needs it. She really is doing great.

Our attention focuses on getting her to eat. My dad and I find a pretty good rhythm working together with Alex. However, we spend hours and hours trying to coerce her into eating. We order everything we can think of from the patient menu. We ask people we barely know to bring her favorite foods in from area restaurants. We even manage to get her all-time favorite: black bean soup from Panera Bread. It seems that her taste buds have changed as a result of her brain damage. She had eaten so healthily before her stroke. Now the only thing that entices her is chocolate.

We are involved in our routine of trying to get Alex to focus on the TV while we try to get her to drink a power drink. She just sorts of zones out. I can't get her to respond to me. I think she is ignoring me to avoid eating. I feel annoyed until I see drool coming out her mouth. She starts to shake—a seizure. We press the nurse button and get help quickly. One of our favorite nurses is on duty. She is quick to help Alex but the shaking and drooling don't stop. The seizure seems like it lasts forever. It is horrifying. The nurses and doctors can't get an IV in her to deliver the medicine. Her veins are still such a mess. I think we are losing her.

Friday, April 2, 2010 9:05 PM

Alex had a grand mal seizure this afternoon. It lasted somewhere between five and eight minutes. She is on IV meds now and seems stable. Enough already.

—Juli

I am scared half to death. How can we contemplate transferring Alex to another hospital for rehab? We will just have to stay here forever. Alex is too unstable. Was the seizure from dropping her medication or was it from her brain bleed? We can't know for sure. We bring her medication level back up and just go on with life. I don't think my heart rate returns to normal until the next day.

My Sister Comes and Brings Her Silliness with Her

Alex does not have another seizure after that first awful one. Eventually, we stop worrying about it and move to focusing on rehab with full force. Part of what we need to do in rehab is help

Alex stay motivated. What motivates her is interesting. She will work very hard for little trinkets, such as little plastic animals. We can get her to try to stand or to try to eat something if we bribe her with a trinket. What works even better is to bribe her with trips to the in-hospital beautician. She just loves it there. The beautician puts nail polish on her fingernails or trims her hair and Alex is so happy. These sorts of things were not important to Alex before the brain bleed.

My sister, Marni, comes to visit. Marni is just silly. It is an interesting contrast when you know that she is also a successful family law attorney so I guess she isn't silly all the time. She is silly with Alex, which is exactly what we need. I am in a rut of nagging Alex to get her to eat and to keep her participating in her rehab activities. My sister achieves even better results without nagging but by being silly instead. It is tough to explain but it works. For example, when my dad and I look through the menu, we try eggs in addition to French toast and we think we are being creative. When my sister arrives, she orders ice cream and chocolate to top the pancakes. That works much better.

Similarly, when Marni wants Alex to try to stand longer, she tells Alex she will make a fish face for the entire time that Alex stands and Alex is motivated to stand longer. She even gets our dad, who is almost bald, to wear a blond wig with her while Alex is getting her hair cut to get Alex to allow the beautician to trim her hair near her incision. What I learn from this is that I don't have to nag. I can have fun with Alex with even better results. This is an epiphany for me; it changes the way I work with Alex from now on. I knew this before as I always use humor in teaching but I had lost perspective as I worked so closely with Alex. I needed a reminder that the environment plays an important role in learning. Alex needs an environment that is positive and fun. It seems that everyone who comes to support Alex makes an important contribution to her recovery.

Friday, April 9, 2010 2:13 AM

I'm sorry it has been so long since my last update. Living in a hospital room 24/7 makes for a surprisingly busy life.

I am happy to report that Alex continues to improve. I hadn't realized just how much until I reread an email I sent just three weeks ago when Jessica and my mom came to visit. At that time, Alex had not yet spoken or sat up. I wrote to say that we were fairly sure she had smiled.

As of today, Alex is beginning to speak in short sentences. She uses a combination of words, phrases, and gestures to communicate and she is getting her point across better and better. She gets frustrated when we are slow on the uptake but we are working on it. We can see that her ability to reason is improving, although she gets confused with some concepts that seem surprising to me. For example, she doesn't know her own body parts. I imagine we will see more of that the more she is able to communicate. However, I continue to be blown away by how much she understands. She is now able to select the correct buttons in the elevator and she has written her name (left-handed).

She is getting stronger physically. She still cannot move her right arm or leg; however, she has learned to transition herself from her wheelchair to the bed and back with very little support. Last night she was even able to sit up in the middle of the bed and hold herself that way unassisted for a few minutes.

Her right ankle and foot was casted yesterday. Her ankle was stretched slightly before casting. This will be repeated every few days for the next two weeks or so. There is some hope the cast will stretch her ankle contracture somewhat, making surgery to release her Achilles tendon unnecessary.

Our biggest news is that Alex's feeding tube was removed yesterday. This is a trial to see if she will eat and drink enough on her own. She takes her pills without a problem so we are safe there. We will need to record every bite and sip over the next few days. She will have another feeding tube placed if necessary. We hope to avoid that. It is just amazing to have Alex without any tubes going into her. I am attaching two pictures my sister took of Alex. One with the feeding tube and Alex's beautiful smile and one taken just after the feeding tube was removed. Marni left yesterday; she was a huge help this week. We are back to my dad and me as Alex's onsite support crew.

The plan at this point is to transfer to an inpatient rehab center in Georgia or Florida in two and a half weeks. We will likely be there for one to two months before moving to an outpatient facility in Orlando and living at home. That is as far as I can project at this point and it is all quite tentative. Marc is researching/

visiting the inpatient rehab centers, as are Alex's doctors here. It is a tough decision. We need to balance the benefits of being close to home so that Alex will have visitors she knows with the specific services the facilities offer. It will be difficult to leave this hospital. Alex is their miracle. Doctors and nurses continue to check in on Alex even after their services are no longer required to see her excellent progress and to share in our celebrations of Alex's victories. The doctors here know her story so intimately and are motivated for her to succeed. The sense of security we feel here is not minor. While it is tempting to stay, all involved know the importance of beginning the process of going home.

Love,
Juli

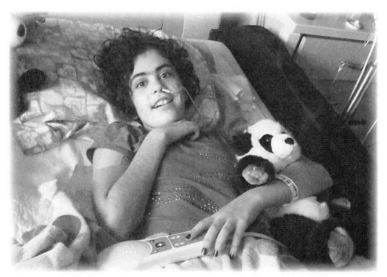

Alex with feeding tube.

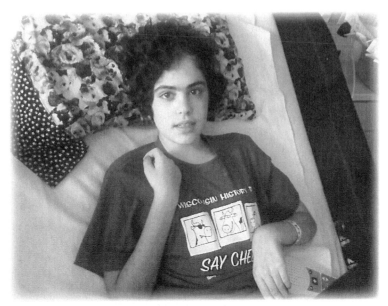

Alex without feeding tube.

We are getting closer to home. It is wonderful, exciting, and terrifying. It helps to reread emails I send to see Alex's progress.

Choosing the correct rehab facility is tough. As always, we want the very best. Determining what that is seems difficult. Our choices are limited. There aren't many children with this sort of issue. Most places don't take children. We will have to make do with the choices we have.

Leaving Our Village

Wednesday, April 14, 2010 11:27 PM

We've finally made a decision regarding our next step. Alex, my dad, and I are flying to Florida tomorrow to transfer to a pediatric inpatient rehab program in a hospital on the west coast of Florida. It is one of two accredited pediatric rehab programs in Florida. Marc, my mom, and Jessica checked it out last Saturday and they were pleased. We are looking forward to getting closer to home, family, and friends. We are anxious about leaving Dr. Alden and making the trip. The week leading to this decision was extremely hectic. I'm sorry to anyone I did not call or email back. I'm sure there were several such instances. It is difficult to describe just how busy I am here.

We said our thank-yous and good-byes to the pediatric ICU nurses and doctors, the general floor nurses, and of course, Sarah and Dr. Alden. The nurses and child life specialists even had a cake for Alex.

We will leave the hospital at six a.m. tomorrow and we will drive a rental car one and a half hours to the airport. We felt a direct flight would be better and there are none from this area. We will fly from Wisconsin to the west coast of Florida. My mom and Jessica will drive there to pick us up at the airport at three p.m. and bring us to the hospital. The hospital has a bed waiting for Alex. She will likely be in rehab there for two to six weeks. From there we will transition home to begin outpatient rehab.

While there we hope to have people Alex knows visit her. We need to find out about policies for visitors and we will need to see how Alex is doing. Too much stimulation is tough on her brain as it continues to heal and we will plan accordingly. Her first visitor will be Marc on Friday. We can't wait.

Love,
Juli

Leaving is terrifying. I am a mess. I am absolutely addicted to Dr. Alden's support. I even have trouble waiting on Sundays for him to go to church before coming to see Alex. How are we going to manage without him? He has been so good to us.

It is the night before we are to leave. Dr. Alden and Sarah meet with my dad and me. Typically when we meet together, we all sit around in Alex's room. This time Dr. Alden asks the child life specialist to stay with Alex and we meet in a room down the hall. That seems strange.

Once Dr. Alden starts talking I know why we are not with Alex. He has determined what happened to cause the brain bleed. It was an accident.

In a sense I am stunned by the news but in another way he is telling me something I think I knew all along. It was the resident's fault. The resident who had told me that he thought Alex's spasms were psychogenic when we were first transferred to the ICU. I hadn't liked him since then. He assisted Dr. Alden with Alex's surgery to get her DBS, the surgery that had gone so badly.

During that surgery, Dr. Alden had needed to pass a shunt from Alex's DBS to her neck to connect to the battery in her chest. The shunt had not been easy to pass. The resident assisted by passing a shunt from her neck up toward the DBS. This should have been a minor routine assist. Dr. Alden tells us the resident missed and punctured Alex's brain. He wiped out the left hemisphere of her brain and caused her to have a stroke.

This is a lot to take. On the one hand, we were at the end of our rope when we brought Alex to this place. Now, she is not in pain. She is no longer spasming. She is improving every day. However, she cannot read, move her right leg, move her right arm. She can't even pee on her own. She has half a brain.

Dr. Alden says that one reason her spasms might not have returned is due to the trauma to her brain caused by the accident. When she had surgery to place the DBS, we were out of options. The DBS would be turned on immediately to begin to control her spasms. After the stroke, we hadn't turned on the DBS; there had been no need, as the spasms did not return. Had this awful accident actually saved her life by stopping the spasms that were killing her? Had it been a stroke of luck? We will never know. Our time in this hospital is complicated and it is a package deal. We cannot separate one thing from another.

A psychologist once told me of a Greek philosopher who alluded to the idea that life is ever changing like a river. At first that doesn't sound quite accurate—until you think about rivers. As the water flows, the rivers are constantly changing. Even if you stay in the same location, the river has changed. That is Alex—changed. Every part of what happened to her influenced her change. We cannot go back in time to the Alex we brought to this hospital. I'm not sure that would be a better choice anyway. That Alex was out of hope and in so much pain. This new Alex is the epitome of hope.

We are beginning a new chapter of her life, one of healing and hope. We are taking a big step toward bringing her home. First, we have to get to Florida.

PART IV: HOMEWARD BOUND

19

Flying to Florida

The trip offers more than we can handle in many ways. We say our good-byes early Thursday morning and my dad and I take the elevator down to the garage under the hospital and wheel Alex to the rental car. My dad parked the car right next to the exit door. What a shock when I see it. In keeping with his tendency to be frugal, Dad rented a compact car rather than a luxury car or minivan, not thinking about how Alex will get in or out. How do we get Alex in the car?

"I can't get the door to stay open far enough so Alex can transition from the wheelchair into the backseat."

"Try the front seat, Juli."

"It's better but it still won't work. What are we going to do?"

"Get her as close as you can, then lift her, I'll move the wheelchair and you can turn her. I'll come behind you and guide her head."

"Okay, hurry—it's cold! I can't believe they didn't teach us how to do this before we left. Alex, you have to bend down, like you're reaching for the ground. That's it—Dad, watch her head!" We make it. I feel abandoned. Nobody at the hospital discussed how to get Alex into a car; we were all thinking of too many other obstacles relative to this transition. I feel panicked before we even leave the hospital garage.

We start on our way after a fair amount of maneuvering to get Alex into the car. After an uneventful drive, we get Alex out of the car without too much trouble. I stay with her in the airport ticketing area while my dad returns the rental car. I feel unexpectedly exposed and nervous. I am surprised how strange it feels to be alone with Alex outside of the hospital. I brought her all over the east coast of the United States in a wheelchair prior to her stroke so that isn't it. Everything feels different now. I am afraid to be alone with my own daughter. Once I realize my fear, I fight the feeling away. I refuse to feel that way. She is my daughter and I will handle anything that happens. I feel proud of myself for releasing that feeling. A feeling of panic replaces it before long.

I keep making Alex drink her energy drink, worried she will not have enough calories during the trip. I worry she will feel weak. Eating presents a challenge and I feel certain she will not eat much during this transition. She needs so much strength and endurance for the trip.

All the drinking makes her bladder feel full. She has to pee. She has to pee! Now what? I can't very well lay her down on the floor in the airport terminal and catheterize her. I'm certainly not going to lay her down on the floor of a public bathroom in an airport. That's just disgusting. I can barely get myself to sit on the toilet seat in airport bathrooms. We really aren't prepared for this trip. How could we have gotten into this mess? We need to find a way over this hurdle—quickly.

We find a family restroom so that my dad and I can both go in with Alex. I will need his assistance. At this point I realize we never learned to transfer Alex from her wheelchair to any other toilet than the one in her hospital room, one designed for it. That toilet had a handle and a side guard so Alex wouldn't fall off. My dad, Alex, and I work together well and get Alex onto the toilet without anything falling in, something almost as difficult as getting Alex into the car. Next we need to figure out how to catheterize her. It is difficult to express what this entails. Kneeling down in front of the toilet in a smelly airport bathroom, trying not to think about what I am kneeling on, attempting to catheterize my daughter by basically sticking my hands into the toilet bowl just above the water, and being careful not to touch the inside of the dirty bowl. Is this some kind of sick joke? I have no idea what to do. I feel like I am in surgery with my dad handing me what I need: wipes, catheter, ointment, etc. I try to keep my voice calm and soothing so that Alex won't get panicked but I'm sure she knows how I feel. Apparently, the perceptive part of her brain remained intact. She takes the situation in stride. We even laugh. Our choice is to laugh or cry and we gave up on crying awhile back.

Everything comes out okay and on to the gate we go. Another story to share with the family: catheterizing Alex on an airport toilet. Getting her onto the plane seems easy compared to that. She feels nervous about sending her wheelchair to be loaded onto the plane, indicating her memory of the difficulties related to the trip from Orlando to Wisconsin remains intact. However, this time, all works out with her wheelchair. We are on our way.

Thank goodness she doesn't need to pee during the flight. I can't imagine trying to go through that in an airplane toilet. I think she feels too excited and nervous. The rest of the trip brings no more drama; I become much more comfortable taking care of Alex. However, I look forward to getting settled into the next hospital.

A Very Different Hospital

I feel excited about getting to the next hospital right up until we get there. I feel disappointed and even a bit horrified when I see it. It is old. It seems unorganized and it even seems dirty and so noisy.

They assign Alex to a tiny room on a busy hallway with scaffolding outside her window. The hospital is being renovated and it definitely needs it. Her window has a metal grate across it. It looks across at another wall anyway; no natural light makes its way into her room. Her ancient bathroom verges on the point of being gross. This assessment is based on a comparison of numerous bathrooms in numerous hospitals. The small bathroom makes it impossible for her to get into it. The wheelchair won't fit. She uses the toilet to defecate. She needs to be able to get to a toilet. We will not go back to diapers just because the room doesn't accommodate our needs.

The hallway has stuff everywhere. Honestly, I feel like we've entered a third-world country. The last hospital was brand-new—beautiful, clean, and organized. All the equipment had places for storage. The bathrooms were large enough to accommodate wheelchairs. We had gotten spoiled. Now we want to go back.

I complain profusely. I will be embarrassed by my behavior later when I am looking back on this. But outside stimuli affect Alex's mood and ability to function. Her dark and dingy room will not be beneficial. The noise in the hallway will be a problem. There is so much traffic in that area. I tell the rehab director that the situation is not acceptable. I say that if I had known that the conditions were this deplorable we would have gone elsewhere. Marc, my mom, and Jessica visited this hospital when we were making plans to transition to a rehab facility closer to home but they toured a different area of the hospital.

The area they saw was bright and less chaotic. Had the rehab nurse purposefully misled us?

As it turns out, the area they had shown my family is full. Somehow they manage to have us moved to that hallway anyway after I complain so profusely. I'm sure that it is no small feat. They do everything in their power to accommodate us. We move to a hallway on the regular pediatric floor but devoted to rehab patients, patients with brain injuries.

The room has a bathroom we can get her wheelchair into; however, the bathroom is shared with another room. Alex has to share a bathroom with a teenage boy! I blow my lid once again when I find out. Is this for real?

Perspective is an important thing to keep as you go through life. It seems that just as you need it most, it can slip away. As it turns out, this hospital works out fine and sharing the bathroom is no big deal. The adult rehab facility connected to the hospital is brand-new and amazing. Eventually, Alex is able to use it but she continues to stay in the very old pediatric wing of the hospital. The therapists at this hospital are true problem solvers. They find ways to help Alex accomplish significant goals. They are a big part of Alex's success in this stage of recovery.

CHARADES (BY JESSICA DIXON)

Alex is coming to Florida finally! I will get to see Mom! Grandma and I leave to go to the airport. This time no false visions of a happy normal family life enter my head. I am too mature for that nonsense now. I know the facts and I am not going to let my guard down. It is better to be hopeless now than let down later. I still wonder how she is doing and how Mom is handling my "baby sister." Still guarded I can't contain my excitement for more than five minutes. She maybe isn't the Alex I know and love, but I still love her even when she is stuck in her baby-like ways.

When I get there Mom and the "less-of-a-baby Alex" meet Grandma and me. Mom is seemingly happy and less-of-a-baby Alex is too. She is a lot better! To hear her voice I want to step down and be a little sister again, but I cannot. I still need to carry on this role. Alex would do the same for me.

In the car after picking them up, I reach a big improvement in Alex's and my relationship. It is also an important step to keeping (or gaining) my mental health. I stop thinking of Alex as "baby Alex" but as my sister Alex. It feels weird to think of her not as baby Alex or new Alex but Alex. I don't reach this on my own. In fact Alex leads me to it. Her bubbly personality makes me feel, well, like part of a family again. Not part of a three-quarter family, but as part of a whole new one. It doesn't even feel new, it feels familiar.

In the car Alex talks and talks. I really like it this way. It feels amazing. Not the "amazing" people normally use but the breathtaking, "once in a lifetime" one. I know I will keep this moment in my memory forever. Alex has a lot of wrong grammar, but I get what she means and that is good enough. She gets stuck on a word and we all play a version of charades. She explains or acts out what she means and we have to guess the word. The longer it takes or the more wrong answers we get, the angrier she gets. When we all can't get what she wants to say, something astonishing happens. Her voice changes and she sounds like her "before voice." In the heat of emotion she doesn't struggle to break the barrier but goes through it. I whisper that into Mom's ear as we pull up to the hospital. We never do figure out what that word is.

We all check in and get settled in the hospital. I can visibly see Grandma struggle not to correct Alex's grammar. Grandma the reading teacher is always fixing my grammar. Trust me, I need it. I can't spell, and I always say "me and Alex" not "Alex and I." She must be dying to correct Alex. It is already obvious Grandma will be a big part of teaching Alex to communicate better.

It was a long day. It is time to go to the Ronald McDonald House across the road from the hospital. Grandma, Grandpa, and I walk there, leaving Mom and Alex at the hospital. When we walk into the place, a lady appears. She shows us our room and takes me to the toy room. The toy room is filled with shelves that are covered with boxes of popular toys for boys and girls. They give them out to the sick children and their siblings. I pick out a box of cute plastic animals with magnets on their feet that attach them to the little stuff they come with. Alex and I played with toys like these often when Alex was sick. The one I pick out is a lemonade stand scene.

The room is nice with two beds and a window looking out on a big oak tree below. Grandma and Grandpa sleep on one bed and I sleep on the other. I often take meds to help me sleep but even those can't save me from what happens next. Both of them snore. Grandpa snores like a bulldozer and Grandma breathes loudly, then lets out an occasional snort. It is snore heaven. Unfortunately snore heaven isn't sleep heaven for me. All I can say is it is a loud night.

I come up to see Alex and Mom every weekend and I leave for school on Sunday. It is a bright time. Alex and I play with the little animals. She likes the boxer dog. It looks like our neighbor's dog and she has a plastic one just like it at home. I think she really wants to come home. She still keeps a picture of Panda on her table.

Alex gets mixed up with names and colors. We get in a line and she says our names. We do that today. I am first, Dad is second, and Mom is third with Grandma and Grandpa behind her. She calls me Jessica, she calls Dad, well, Dad, and calls Mom Grandpa. We all crack up. Grandpa is bald on the top of his head and Mom has a long mane of hair. We have to explain this to Alex and she joins in laughing.

Alex is going home soon. Alex's spark finally lit and her eyes have a familiar twinkle. We didn't just get Alex back. We got the real Alex back.

●●

20

Leaving Alex

I keep my career going throughout Alex's journey. It is important to my sanity as well as to our finances. I continue to write articles for professional journals. I made considerable contributions as an author of an elementary school mathematics textbook series from Alex's hospital room. I even Skyped into meetings and dissertation defenses from the ICU. It is a bit surreal but it works. However, I let pass several opportunities in favor of staying by Alex's side. I find it hard to let go of one particular opportunity.

I was asked to give a presentation during a luncheon at the annual meeting of the National Council of Supervisors of Mathematics. It is a big deal. There will likely be about 1,500 people at the lunch. I would need to go for the lunch and then I could come right back to Alex. The presentation will only last forty-five minutes. The only catch? We are in Florida and the meeting is in San Diego. Skype just won't do for this one.

Dr. Alden and Sarah knew about my profession and had asked me about how I was handling things during my time in Wisconsin. During one of these conversations, I told them about the invitation to give this talk. They both urged me to go. They said that Alex would be fine at the hospital and with my mom. They worried I would come to regret letting this opportunity pass. After considerable internal struggle and several long conversations with my family and friends, I choose to go.

I will need to fly in to San Diego the night before my presentation and then take the red-eye home after my talk. I will be gone for just over twenty-four hours. Alex will need to pee while I am gone. That is my job and I don't let anyone else near her to do it. She has already endured too much when people tried to catheterize her without success. Who will catheterize her? My mom doesn't mind taking on the responsibility but Alex doesn't want her to take my place.

I begin to realize how important it is for me to go. Alex and I are too attached. I teach my mom what to do despite Alex's objections and make plans for my trip. I prepare for my presentation during the evenings prior to my trip after Alex falls asleep. Marc brings me a suit from home to wear in San Diego. We will make this work.

Alex does fine but I feel like a mess the entire time I am gone. I must call my mother a hundred times during a twenty-four-hour period. Alex is all I can think about. I have focused solely on her for so long I can barely carry on a conversation about anything else. I'll never forget standing on a stage in front of 1,500 people. I prepared to give a talk about mathematics education. All I want to do is to tell the participants about my daughter— how she is working so hard to take back her life, how she has such a great attitude. How she struggled to get people to believe in her for two years and then the unimaginable happened but still she survived and is fighting to regain what she lost. Nothing else seems important. What am I even doing here? It takes all I have to stick with the talk I planned. Will I ever truly return to my professional life as I knew it before? Do I even want that life back?

I feel so happy to get back to the hospital and so proud of how Alex and my mom managed. From this point on, I slowly begin taking on a little more work responsibility. I leave the hospital for a few days at a time to go to a county someplace in Florida and provide professional development for the teachers there. I attend graduation at my university and hood a doctoral student who defended her dissertation and completed her degree while I was with Alex in the hospital. It is tough to be away from Alex but also refreshing. I take the opportunity to begin focusing on things outside of the cocoon I have created around Alex. It is an important phase in our recovery process. It might have been easier to stay single-minded, only focusing on Alex's immediate needs, but I don't think it would have been better for either one of us. My mom and dad step in for me when I am gone. My dad stays in the Ronald McDonald House and my mom stays with Alex. On weekends, they go back to their home on the east coast of Florida and Marc and Jessica take their place at the Ronald McDonald House. Family plays an important role in Alex's recovery. As Alex continues to heal, she and Jessica continue to renegotiate their relationship. This will be an ongoing process.

Family Time

It is nice to be close to home, just two hours away. On weekends, Marc, Jessica, Alex, and I spend every waking moment together.

Saturday, April 17, 2010 9:10 AM

Good morning,

We are settled into our new digs in Florida in the pediatric rehab area of the hospital. A very old building but we have a beautiful riverside view.

The child life specialist brought a Wii cart into our room yesterday to use for the weekend and Alex and Jessica played tennis, bowling, and baseball for well over an hour! Times like this help me to envision our transition home and back to a life as a family.

It took Alex a bit of time to get accustomed to using her left hand to play but she is getting better and better. She still has no use of her right arm so activities like this are excellent, and that is why this Wii is part of her rehab experience.

For now, Alex is getting casts on her right leg. They are replaced every few days to stretch her ankle. We are working on every strategy to get her to eat as she is fifteen pounds underweight and nothing tastes good to her. She is learning to help with daily living tasks like feeding herself, getting dressed, washing, getting from her bed to her wheelchair, etc. She is in therapy to help her to walk (there is a possibility she will be able to do so). Speech therapy is focused on speaking and understanding. She is getting easier to understand; she communicates better each day. She is still quite limited but she does get her point across.

The weekend afternoons will be the best time for visitors but we've been told to be careful not to overwhelm her. She is kept extremely busy during the week and she has therapies on weekend mornings. I have no idea how long we will be here. It could be two weeks or two months . . . .

Take care,
Juli

While weekdays are full of hours and hours of therapy, weekends consist of free time—a lot of free time. It is sometimes difficult to fill the hours.

Previously right-handed, Alex quickly becomes adept at doing things with her left hand. It is impressive. Alex becomes the champion at bowling on the Wii. It is tough for Jessica. On the one hand, she is working hard to be the "big sister." She lets Alex have her way and win at so many things. On the other hand, when Alex actually does something better than Jessica, Jessica finds it difficult to take. She truly is learning to take the role of the big sister. However, Alex was such a good big sister before that Jessica never realized that not getting your own way all the time is part of the job description.

We go on outings to the Ronald McDonald House. The volunteers go out of their way to make people feel welcome. There are always donated treats in the kitchen like cupcakes and brownies. There are activities occasionally, like making crafts. The community living spaces are comfortable with soft couches, warm light from lamps, books for borrowing, and games to use.

The House is within walking distance so we can just wheel Alex there in her wheelchair. One of Alex's favorite things at the Ronald McDonald House is the big aquarium. There is a huge slug in the aquarium, though it is actually a sea hare. Every time we come here we look for the slug. She wants to take it home. I think Alex remembers the word "slug" before she can remember her own name.

It is strange to think she cannot even remember her own name. There must be a strategy that can help her. As an educator, I know the best ways to help someone to remember something is to help him or her to understand it and to provide some sort of emotional connection. There is nothing to understand about a name so I have to go with the emotional connection.

There is a fairly steep ramp that we use to get on and off the Ronald McDonald House property. Every time Alex is wheeled down the ramp she says, "Ahhhhhhhhhhh!" She loves it. I use this emotion to help her remember her name. As she wheels down the ramp I say, "Use this to remember your name—your name is AAAAAAAAAlex." It works, but for the next three months, every time she tells someone her name, she says, "AAAAAAlex."

There is also a piano at the Ronald McDonald House, an old upright against the wall in one of the living rooms. It is amazing to me that Alex can remember how to play songs she played as a child—simple songs like "Twinkle, Twinkle Little Star," but also parts of songs she was working on with her piano teacher before her stroke, like "The Pink Panther." The music is just there in her brain. Maybe because that part of her brain is not damaged, music continues to take a place of importance. We capitalize on that to help her to regain language. The more we can get Alex to sing, the more practice she has at forming words in her mouth and the more she is reminded of the speed and rhythm of speaking. Certain songs are more important to Alex than others; some evolve into theme songs.

The Climb

One song that has particular significance to Alex as a theme song is Miley Cyrus's "The Climb," which reflects her perception of where she is and what she will need to do to get her life back. The song talks about needing to be strong to overcome hurdles, to climb mountains. It talks about the importance of the climb.

She is working so hard. She still performs for rewards but as time goes on she forgets to ask for them. The rewards serve to push her forward when her performance does not provide the intrinsic motivation she needs. As she improves, the rewards are less important. Her own improvement provides sufficient motivation. She truly is focused on the climb and feels proud of her journey.

She spends one to one and a half hours in each daily session of physical therapy (PT), occupational therapy (OT), and speech therapy. The goal of PT is to transition her from her wheelchair to a walker to a cane. We think this goal is too good to be true. How will she ever be able to walk again with only a cane to support her?

Part of the process of being able to walk again has to do with getting her heel down. It still does not touch the floor when she tries to stand on her right foot. Her foot has been pointed for so long that even though we can now stretch her foot and it will actually move—whereas before the stroke we could not stretch it at all—it is still somewhat pointed.

We continue to use serial casts to stretch her Achilles tendon. The casts are a pain. Alex finds it hard to maneuver with the cast. She cannot make her right leg move by just using her brain so when she wants to reposition it she has to lift it with her left arm. With the added weight of the cast, she has more to lift. The casts also gets so dirty, and I mean really dirty. She gets a new cast every three to five days that stretches her foot a few degrees farther each time.

Alex continues to struggle with eating. She gags and vomits frequently. It seems that within one day of getting each new cast she vomits on it. It is disgusting, especially since a large part of her diet consists of a red energy drink. We are getting accustomed to her cast almost always having a red tint to it.

Alex's room has two hospital beds and I sleep in one of them. We place an upright chair between them—there is just enough room. Alex sits on the chair to eat. Getting her in the chair and ready to eat is a production, especially with the heavy cast on her leg. I push the tray table in front of her. I sit in a chair on the other side of the tray table facing her.

"Alex, you have to eat, please eat. . . . I will give you another prize from your reward box if you eat three more bites. . . . You know you need to eat so your brain will continue to heal. . . . If you don't eat you're going to get a feeding tube!" Nothing works and we are constantly teetering on the verge of needing another feeding tube. It will be such a step backward to get one that I make it a major mission to keep her fed. Much of our days continue to revolve around mealtime. Alex tells me she just can't eat more, she can't take another bite or another sip even though she has eaten so little. I push her, relying on my gut. My gut is not always reliable. All too often, Alex takes that one extra bite and then vomits it and everything else all over her tray, her clothes, her cast, and me. It's not pretty. She cannot move her body in a coordinated, controlled, or fast enough fashion to avoid making a mess. She feels bad when it happens but she also makes sure to let me know she warned me.

She handles the casts like she handles everything. She has such a great attitude. She will just do anything to succeed. Often she sleeps with a cast on her leg and a brace on her hand to stretch her hand. She does so without complaining.

She has so much to learn. She needs energy for so many different areas: working on stretching her right foot, walking, using her right hand, eating, taking over her daily living responsibilities with her left hand, writing, reading, speaking, and so on. With so much to work on, some support personnel she encounters lose sight of how smart she is. That hurts her more than anything.

Phalanges

Alex begins receiving hospital/homebound instruction while at this hospital. Her teachers have quite a challenge. Alex can't read or write at all and she can barely speak. Though bright, she doesn't seem to remember anything she was taught in school. She has lifetime memories like playing with her sister, vacations, holidays, and family time. However, she doesn't seem to be able to recall much about social studies, science, or mathematics. Every once in awhile she will recall something and apply it in such a way that she just blindsides you with her intelligence.

While she cannot function like a typical twelve-year-old, she certainly doesn't want to be treated like a baby. Her hospital/homebound teacher makes the fatal error of treating Alex like a baby. It is understandable but not acceptable.

She brings Alex Scooby Doo playing cards to use during her lesson. To keep with the theme she brings Scooby Doo snacks as well. The teacher, proud of her themed lesson idea, shares her plans with us. This appalls Alex; she feels like a baby and I can tell she is waiting to pounce but I don't know how or when.

Ms. Louise, her teacher, begins a lesson on naming body parts, a topic with which Alex struggles. Using a tone of voice one might use with a young child she says, "Alex, this is the nose." She points to the nose on the drawing of a human body. "This is the mouth . . . this is the hand. . . . What are these?" She points to the fingers.

Alex looks her in the eyes and says with considerable strength, "Phalanges." Determined to put the teacher in her place, Alex pulls the scientific name for fingers from some place in her brain. The teacher doesn't know how to respond. She is absolutely amazed. That is how Alex works. She amazes people and draws people in to want to commit everything they have to her journey. She will also take you down if you don't treat her the way she believes she should be treated.

As soon as she leaves the session with Ms. Louise, she says, "Don't like her. Thinks me baby. Not going back." My mother and I are not sure how to react. We suggest that she share her concerns with the neuropsychologist. This provides a good opportunity for Alex to prepare to deal with people in the future who are misguided regarding her intelligence based on how she presents herself. We see this as an important step toward the possibility of independence some day.

She takes every opportunity to learn and my mother and I capitalize on her motivation. I don't know what we would have done if our backgrounds hadn't included being elementary school teachers. We are teaching every grade from preschool to sixth grade simultaneously. We use everything we have ever learned as classroom teachers to help Alex rebuild her cognitive skills.

Alex can't get her colors down. She knows the color names but she can't match them properly to their actual colors. We use dry-erase markers and write the color names in the associated colors on every surface possible in her hospital room. We cover the whiteboard in her room, we write them on mirrors. We get colored construction paper and write the color names on the corresponding colored paper. We connect the color name to everything we touch. "Alex, here is your red toothbrush. What color is your toothbrush? Red. Now put on your purple T-shirt. What color is your T-shirt?" My mother and I say the same things and use the same strategies; there is consistency regardless of who stays with her because it is always my mother or me. It takes her months to relearn her colors. But she finally does. First she is able to choose the color we request. We say, "Point to the red ball," and she does. Naming the colors comes later. We say, "What color is this ball?" She might say, "Blue," when it is green. We just correct her and have her repeat us. Through repetition and multiple representations, she reconnects that knowledge in her brain. It is fascinating to see how so much of what we talk about as good teaching practices are applicable and even necessary to help Alex relearn. Learning needs to be active—Alex participates rather than just listens—and we have her select the ball rather than have us holding the ball and naming the color. Learning needs to be engaging and relevant; Alex chooses fingernail polish in colors because she cares about fingernail polish. Learning needs to be ongoing and repetitive; everything is labeled and we use every opportunity to reinforce our learning goals. The results are so evident. We use the same process for almost everything we do with her. If our goal is to work on people's names, then we label the people and find ways to use their names constantly. When we focus on body parts, we play games with body parts, buy Mr. and Mrs. Potato Head and play with them, and label our own body parts. We use repetition and constant reinforcement.

21

Finding Words

Slowly but surely Alex begins to communicate more. We keep a small dry-erase board with us everywhere we go. She finds words by using as many cues as possible. Sometimes she can think of the first letter sound of the word but not the word. When she can remember the letter sound, she writes that letter on the whiteboard and makes the letter sound and often the word will come to her. Sometimes she can even come up with the first few letters. It is as though she has an image of the word in her mind even though she can't name the letters.

It seems strange that she can begin to write letters, that she knows the sounds in many cases, but that she can't name the letters. Helping Alex to find the words she needs to communicate is like a never-ending game of charades. It is difficult for everyone when we don't guess well. She just points and says, "This, this, this!" with so much frustration in her voice. She cannot just walk over to what she means and show us because she is not yet mobile. She persists. If we spend the day without success in determining what she is trying to communicate, she will often wake up the next morning having come up with another way to try to get at it.

Each night my mom or I lay out Alex's clothes for the next day. The occupational therapist helps Alex learn to dress using one arm. One evening my mother forgets to put out Alex's socks. Alex cannot remember the word "socks" but spends thirty minutes pointing to the suitcase across the room saying, "That, that!" My mother can't figure out what she means. The first thing Alex says to her the next morning is "Sock!" Had she dreamt about that one word all night?

The complex nature of the brain becomes more and more obvious as we continue to work with Alex. She still can't read out loud. However, she can look at a hospital menu and often point to what she wants to order on the menu (not that she will actually eat it when it arrives).

She can't follow more than one direction at a time. For example, her speech therapist asks her to point to the picture of the ball then point to the picture of the dog and she can only point to the ball. After the therapist reads her a short passage Alex gets most of the listening comprehension questions wrong. She cannot seem to make sense of what is read to her. I just hate these times because the questions seem so simple. However, she is still able to reason. She remembers how to play tic-tac-toe. My mom plays it with her so often that Alex eventually gets bored. My mom asks the neuropsychologist if Alex might be able to handle more challenging games. The psychologist says to try. Before long Alex is beating my mom at checkers. She continues to surprise us.

A Giant Step toward Independence

It is early in May, and a welcome surprise comes when I am catheterizing Alex. Alex and I have the routine down. I get Alex ready by having her lie down in her bed on a waterproof mat with her pants down. I get all the materials I need and put them within reach of Alex. She then hands me what I need. Today I get Alex on to the waterproof mat and turn away from Alex to get what I need. Alex calls my name quite excitedly. I turn around to see Alex just peeing everywhere like a baby boy on a changing table—the most welcomed bedwetting I've ever experienced. Alex can pee! It shocks her as much as me. What a relief. This is a major step toward the idea that Alex might one day be able to live independently. It also opens up more freedom for Alex to do things without my mom or me.

The therapists start taking the rehab kids on field trips once per week. It is quite a sight to see a group of adolescents in wheelchairs with significant brain injuries get loaded on a hospital bus to go on an outing with their therapists. The group, made up of girls and boys, represents several ethnicities with ages ranging from about age ten to age seventeen. Such different circumstances brought them together, from illnesses to brain tumors to car accidents. In many instances we have no idea what caused the child's brain injury. Some of the children seem to have no relatives with them. The nurses take these children under their wings. They keep the children with them at the nurses' station during times when there are no therapy sessions.

One particularly rough-looking teenage boy with tattoos all over his arms is often at the nurses' station. He reacts to Alex and my father in the same way every time he sees them. He sort of drawls, "Whassup, girl?" to Alex and, "Whassup, Grandpa?" to my father. It becomes a running joke with our family. Every time my dad walks into Alex's hospital room she says, "Whassup, Grandpa?" and laughs and laughs.

Parents are not allowed to go on the field trips. It is the only time Alex is without a family member. I feel like my heart is being torn out every time I watch the bus drive away with Alex. I can't breathe easily until she comes back a few hours later. She does fine. The kids go to the aquarium, the mall, to get ice cream, and to the grocery store. By the time Alex goes to the grocery store, she is walking with a four-prong cane.

First Steps without a Wheelchair

Alex slowly regains strength. She works extremely hard during physical therapy and her therapist accepts nothing less. She is determined to get Alex walking—a slow process. At first Alex just stands. Then she is hung from the ceiling in a body harness to get accustomed to the mechanics of walking without having to hold her weight. Eventually she uses this contraption on a treadmill holding more and more of her own weight. She hates this part of therapy. She gets the worst wedgies. It is worth it—or at least I think so, though I'm fairly sure Alex doesn't agree. I imagine her walking, standing up from her wheelchair and walking to me, walking her dog, walking in school. It is such a great dream; seeing her standing, even if suspended from the ceiling in a harness, makes the dream seem possible.

Sunday, May 9, 2010 9:45 AM

Good morning,

So I'm sending this update on Mother's Day because recently I have come to feel that every day is Mother's Day. Alex continues to make improvements every single day. She is determined to talk and walk again. She seems to acknowledge somewhere in her mind that she may not get the use of her arm back completely but she does stretch it on her own throughout the day just the same. She can now use her left arm to pull her right arm up over her head.

Alex is remembering more words on her own and she is still so pleased with herself every time she gets one right. She can hear when she says them wrong and that is fantastic. For example, if she says giraffe instead of tiger, she knows she is wrong if she wants to say tiger. She is also getting better at writing words with her left hand on a whiteboard from the image she holds in her mind. My colleagues at UCF made a collection and purchased Alex an iPad, which should be quite useful. Alex is also using more and more sentences. She used to speak in grunts, then with just one word, but now she uses sentences quite frequently. Her speech therapist is thrilled, as are we.

Alex can now stand and transition from the wheelchair to the bed with no assistance. She can also stand holding on to a rail for more than five minutes on her own. She is making the movements of walking on a treadmill while supported from above with a harness. Her PT believes she will walk with some assistive device and minor support from a person before she leaves the rehab hospital. We are hopeful.

This is all great and her therapists and doctors continue to be amazed by her. I am both thankful for where we are and hopeful for where we are going. Jessica continues to be very supportive in this crazy life she finds herself. She is so reflective and accepting. I am honored to be their mother today and every day.

Enjoy the day. I know I will.

Love,
Juli

Eventually Alex begins using a walker. This is a bit tough because she can't hold the walker with both hands. Her right hand is not useful at all. We use a tall walker and we strap her right arm onto the walker to keep it in place. It works—a huge step, so to speak.

She finally begins using a four-prong cane toward the end of her stay at the hospital. A four-prong cane is a cane on a somewhat stable base. It is more stable than a regular cane and it can stand on its own but it is still a cane you hold onto with one hand. Alex gets strong. She walks up and down stairs with assistance. It amazes me to see her walk. She uses a brace like her old Scooby Doo brace to keep her right foot in position. Except this brace is not in a ridiculously pointed position, but instead in a position a normal leg could accommodate while walking. It is covered in butterflies—she has gone from a picture of Scooby Doo on the back of her brace to butterflies. I can't know if this change in preference is strictly from the maturing process or from how the stroke has changed Alex's personality. The serial casts work to get her foot in a position very close to where her heel almost touches the ground.

When she finally starts standing on her own, I am amazed at how tall she's gotten—five foot two—two inches taller than me! She has grown and matured. Once she can talk better, she tells us she grew boobies in her coma. She is right! My daughter is experiencing adolescence in a way I never could have imagined—uncharted territory.

Meeting Panda

Alex's puppy also grew while Alex was in a coma. The breeder kept him for a few extra weeks but then it was time to find him a home. Marc's step-step-grandmother lives near the breeder. She is Marc's stepfather's stepmother and a very dear relative to us.

Grannie, as we call her, has always been especially close to our family. The girls and I visited her during summers when they were younger. She loves birds and sometimes she has as many as seven birds living with her. The girls helped her to care for them. Once Alex became ill, we did not have the opportunity to spend much time with Grannie. She appreciates the opportunity to step in to help now. She found a dog sitter to take in our brand-new puppy. The woman took him in and fell in love with him. She sent Alex pictures to the hospital in Wisconsin. When Alex received them, she had me tape the pictures on her wall so she could look at them regularly. She showed them to everyone who visited.

The dog sitter kept him for quite some time but when she had to leave town Grannie took him in. Grannie has one bird and a cat. It is quite a combination. The cat chases Panda and Panda chases the bird. Panda makes it a chaotic house.

Grannie lives about an hour from the rehab hospital. Once we get settled, she brings Panda to the hospital on weekends. The puppy can't go into the hospital so we go out to the hospital grounds and lay a blanket on the grass. We position Alex on the blanket and give her Panda. While sweet to see her finally meet the puppy of her dreams, it also feels a little strange.

Alex had been a dog fanatic. As a child, every lemonade stand she ever had was to make money to support an animal shelter. Every story she ever wrote had a dog as a main character. We expect her to be beside herself with joy when she meets Panda. She isn't.

We realize she has undergone a personality change. She is no longer a "dog lover." She likes Panda but is not overwhelmed with joy by being with him. Marc and I look at each other as we watch her interact with the dog. We share wonder and worry in our expressions.

We continue our visits with Panda as an important distraction from therapy. Eventually the doctors grant us day passes to leave the hospital grounds on weekends. We have to be back by late evening for insurance purposes. Alex cannot miss a night at the hospital or her stay will have to end altogether. On several of these daytime outings, we visit Grannie at her home. It feels strange to be in a house. It has been months since we used a bathroom other than one in a hospital or sat at a dining room table rather than at a table tray in a hospital room. We can sit on a carpeted floor and not worry about who walked on it. It is nice to be in a home.

On other outings we go to the zoo, to the aquarium, and to get Alex's hair cut. People are so nice to Alex, especially hairdressers. In Wisconsin, on the west coast of Florida, and back home in Orlando, hairdressers refuse to take payment for Alex's haircuts. They do so much to make Alex feel better about herself, taking time to assist her in finding a style to hide the scars all over her scalp. What an amazing gift they are able to give Alex. She cares about how she looks and they help her feel better about her appearance. This is particularly important as she prepares to visit her middle school.

22

There's No Ramp!

It is late May 2010, and I just got an email from one of Alex's teachers asking if Alex can attend the awards assembly at her middle school. They plan to give her two awards and the teachers want to be able to present them to her in person. It is difficult to fathom. When she left, she was so articulate. She was in pain and using forearm crutches and a wheelchair but she was so independent. Now she can barely speak; she needs help with everything. I know she won't be able to remember the names of her friends or her teachers, let alone converse with them. How is this going to work?

Alex will need to go to therapy all day, then drive two hours to the assembly. We will need to get back to the hospital that same night due to insurance rules. It will be a late night and a long and emotional day. I discuss it with Alex and she wants to go. Does she realize how different she is now? Does she realize that when she speaks the students and probably the teachers will stare at her? I guess we have to do this at some point—we can't live in this cocoon of people who expect Alex to be this way forever. I check with her therapists and they think it a great idea—I guess it is time to venture out. We are going.

Seeing all the teachers and students overwhelms Alex. I just keep whispering their names in her ear from behind her wheelchair. She handles things beautifully. She just says, "I know you but I don't know your name," over and over again. People seem to be okay with that. I don't think they know what to say to Alex or how to behave around her. They mostly look down at her in the wheelchair, smile, tilt their heads, and tell her how great she looks. She does look great. She is wearing a deep purple short-sleeve shirt with frills down the front. It was *very* difficult to get it on her with how her right arm just hangs there but we did it. It is so much more difficult to put on shirts that aren't stretchy; we need to add that to the tasks the OT works on. It is worth the effort. Alex looks beautiful; she is sitting so tall and her pale skin and dark hair and eyes are a lovely contrast to the deep purple. Everyone seems happy to see her. The teachers know all about what she has gone through from my emails. The students just know she has been struggling. They have been sending her good thoughts the entire time she's been away. Still, they are only sixth graders and it is a lot to take in. I can see them stealing looks at the scar still visible on Alex's head through her short hair. I'm sure they have so many questions that they will ask their teachers and parents when they are out of earshot. I have an urge to explain all Alex has been through and how far she has come but the opportunity doesn't present itself.

The awards Alex receives are for her Odyssey of the Mind team making it to state and for a state-level award for her National History Day project on the Americans with Disabilities Act. While she can walk short distances with a cane, she can only do it with her therapist holding a safety harness around her waist. She uses a wheelchair for the awards assembly.

The assembly is in the gymnasium, which also serves as the auditorium. The students sit on folding chairs lining the gymnasium floor and the parents and other family members fill the bleachers that line the perimeter of the room. A stage has been erected at one end of the gym. Alex's name is called and I wheel her to the stage for her award for her project on the Americans with Disabilities Act. Alex is sitting in her wheelchair at the end of the bleachers, I sit next to her on the first step of the bleachers. As we get closer to the stage it becomes obvious that Alex will not be able to get up on the stage to receive her award. There is no ramp. The administrators are embarrassed and that is a good thing. I hope their feelings of discomfort will help to create change. I wonder how in 2010—so many years after the Americans with Disabilities Act addressed accessibility issues for physical disabilities—there could not be a ramp to get my daughter up on stage?

Alex handles it with grace as I wheel her in front of the stage to get the award. The administrators on stage have to squat down to reach us to place Alex's medal around her neck. She sees the irony in the situation. The stage she encounters to get an award for a project related to accessibility is not accessible. She understands this. Here is another clear indication that I know Alex will be okay.

Going Home

Shortly after the awards assembly, the rehab hospital discharges Alex. Just like when we transitioned from the Wisconsin hospital to this hospital, we are not prepared. Maybe people can never be truly prepared for these sorts of transitions. It is a very difficult time. I call Dr. Alden for advice as I do so often and he says that he will see what he can do. He gets the hospital in Wisconsin to agree to pay for another two weeks of rehab at the rehab hospital in Florida to provide support for Alex. I can only imagine that it is because of the accident during surgery.

I am thrilled. I can't wait to tell the rehab doctor in Florida. I am so excited to hear his reaction because I know this sort of opportunity is unusual. I get the news while I am doing our laundry at the Ronald McDonald House. I don't wait a minute and I call right from the laundry room.

"Did you hear what Dr. Alden got the Wisconsin hospital to offer?"

"Yes. That was very nice of him. He really cares for Alex deeply."

Wait, he doesn't sound excited. This is not going the way I thought it would. "So, are we going to stay two more weeks?"

"I don't think so. It is time for Alex to go home and continue rehab from there."

He is still going to send Alex home! How can he do this? I want to cry and scream at the same time. "I don't agree with your decision. She is doing so well, and she hasn't stopped improving. Two more weeks here will get her much further than if we go home."

"I understand your concern but this is the right decision." He is clearly done discussing this with me.

We aren't ready. I feel so angry about this decision. I still don't understand it. Dr. Alden had been communicating with his hospital since the accident to find ways to support Alex. He had gotten his hospital to pay for the rehab portion of Alex's stay in Wisconsin. Now he has gotten them to agree to pay for two weeks of rehab at this hospital. I'm sure that was no small feat. The rehab doctor won't take it. I don't know if it is because of politics, reporting statistics, or Alex's progress. One way rehab hospitals report their success is by how quickly they provide rehabilitation for their patients. They report the average number of nights patients stay and the lower the number, the better. I imagine that Alex is blowing their average. I don't know if this has anything to do with the decision to send Alex home, but it just doesn't feel right to me. I can't forgive the rehab doctor for this decision but I also can't change his mind. The doctor says it is time to continue rehab at home, but Alex is making such great progress right where she is. How could he do this to us?

Transitioning home proves difficult. How is it that each time we are discharged and sent to the next lower level of support, we find ourselves completely unprepared for the change? Just like I think that architects and engineers should spend a day in a wheelchair in the structures they design, I think that rehab doctors should live through these sorts of transitions with their patients.

PART V:
FINALLY HOME

23

Home Sweet Home

Home sweet home feels anything but sweet. Alex hasn't been alone since before her stroke and we certainly don't feel she is ready to be alone now. We bring a mattress into her room and put it on the floor so Marc can sleep there. We buy a rail to put on the edge of her bed to insure she will not roll out of bed. We also get a shallower box spring to lower the height of her bed so she can get in and out of bed. All of this has to be done so fast so that Alex will be safe. We are exhausted.

All of the bedrooms in our house have carpeting. Alex has not walked or wheeled her wheelchair on carpet during rehab and it is much more difficult than tile or wood floors. We hadn't anticipated this. While we are able to remove the area rugs from the rest of the house, we are not prepared to deal with the carpet. We end up replacing all the carpet in the house with wood floors—not easy to do while we are all in the house. I wish we had thought of it earlier so we could have replaced them before Alex and I came home. I guess we thought we would have more time or maybe we just weren't thinking about the future. I am upset with myself for not being prepared. I guess maybe some of these things, like always anticipating the next obstacle, just aren't so easy.

Even bringing Alex to the bathroom proves difficult. The

bathrooms are so hard to manage with a wheelchair. She can't get to the sinks or the toilets well. Showering is also difficult. We eventually find ways to make this work but it takes effort. We even need to make changes to the type of shampoo dispenser. Alex can't hold a bottle in one hand and poor the shampoo into the other. We install shampoo and conditioner pumps on the shower wall. This is minor, but when we add up all the minor changes, we have some major adjustments to make.

Marc and I are determined to continue Alex's progress toward independence so we buy a baby monitor and place it in her room so we can sleep in ours. It feels strange to sleep together in our own room away from Alex. I feel like a mother of an infant listening to the baby monitor for Alex's breathing to assure me she is all right.

With all we are figuring out at home, we want to make sure Alex's rehab continues outside of our home. We have a terrible time finding rehab appropriate for Alex. Children just don't have strokes. The pediatric facilities don't seem to be able to provide the level of therapy Alex needs and the adult facilities designed for people who had strokes won't take her, although eventually they do. It would be great if we could find therapists who will come to our home but we can't find those either. It takes months to settle in with therapists and a therapy schedule tailored to Alex's needs—wasted months in my mind. This should be part of the transition process. We were told we would receive this and people do try to help us. They make phone calls and give us numbers to call but when we follow their directions the outpatient rehab is not as they indicated. Either the facility has no room for new patients or Alex is too young or too old. The support we are given does not end up being supportive. Once again, people who help transition should try the transitions themselves.

Even with all the issues related to the transition, after a while it feels so good to be home. Alex's friends come to visit. I worry unnecessarily about them finding ways to interact.

Alex's friends Anna and Rebecca visit shortly after our return home. Alex wants to play Cadoo™ by Cranium™, a game that involves a form of charades, acting, drawing, and molding clay. I think it a strange choice—other than the reference to the cranium, a part of Alex receiving considerable attention. Alex can't read the cues, she can't mold clay with one hand, and the game requires she draw. Because her right hand doesn't work, she will need to draw left-handed—something she has not yet mastered to say the least. The girls play in the family room and I observe from the kitchen, pretending to look busy hand-washing dishes normally put in the dishwasher. I'm worried that Anna and Rebecca won't know how to help Alex participate. The girls naturally adapt to Alex's deficits; they read the cue cards to her, allow her extra time to solve the puzzles, and help her find words. Watching a child with aphasia play charades is funny. Alex calls out, "I know it, I know it—I just don't know what it's called." The girls are stumped for ways to help her. They give her a hint using words. They begin asking her to just say what the word starts with and if she gets that she wins. They make sure she wins. I'm worried that the girls are bored by Alex. I find a reason for them to come with me to the next room and I tell them they don't have to feel obligated to stay and hang out with Alex. They seem to truly enjoy their time with her even though she is not the same girl they had known before the stroke; they say they want to stay. Others respond in the same way. Alex never had a large number of friends but those she had stick with her, finding ways to interact within Alex's limitations.

A Thousand Paper Cranes

Remember when Alex was struggling in the ICU and her teachers contacted me to let me know that Alex's classmates wanted to do something to support her to show they cared? I had not known what to say, as we really didn't know how things were going to turn out. We did not want them to have a fundraiser because it seemed too public. What if Alex died or had not been well enough to ever come back home? I would not have been able to face her classmates to tell them the bad news. It was better not to make plans. Alex's teachers understood. These teachers were very close to Alex. Ms. Capp was her sixth-grade gifted advanced geography teacher who had supported her efforts in the National History Day project, bringing the project to Tallahassee so Alex could compete at the state level while in the hospital. That was quite an undertaking. Ms. Poarch, her Odyssey of the Mind coach, helped Alex become part of a team when she started middle school in a wheelchair. She also went on to bring Alex's team to state while Alex was in the ICU.

These teachers understood Alex's classmates' needs to show Alex they cared. Without my knowing, they organized the students and the teachers at the school in folding a thousand paper cranes in honor of the tale that a wish will be granted following the folding of a thousand paper cranes. The students folded them during the months Alex was hospitalized. They wished for Alex to get better and come back to school.

We've been home for one week. Ms. Capp, Ms. Poarch, and Ms. Hunziker, Alex's gifted advanced mathematics teacher, come to our home with the cranes. They carry box after box of large clear plastic storage bins of cranes into the house. Marc is at work, but Jessica, Alex, and I watch in amazement as the teachers deposit the boxes in Alex's room, filling the floor with brightly colored folded wishes. Alex, overwhelmed with emotion, hugs the teachers with her tight one-armed hug, pulling them close. The teachers weep with relief to see Alex again and with pain for losing the articulate student they had mentored, the student who can no longer remember their names but still knows their roles in her life. I have grown accustomed to Alex's limited speech, the more childish tone of her voice, and her paralyzed arm. Her teachers have much to take in; they seem overwhelmed in ways that Alex's friends aren't affected, as if the friends are able to move forward with Alex at face value but adults reflect on what they have lost, comparing Alex to her pre-stroke self. Eventually, they become accustomed to the new Alex and we settle in to a feeling of warm camaraderie. We sit in Alex's bedroom—Alex in her wheelchair, Ms. Poarch and I on her bed, and Ms. Capp and Ms. Hunziker in chairs I bring in from the kitchen. We visit while we string the cranes together with thread. Alex practices using her right hand by trying to grab cranes from the box to then give us to thread. She needs to bend her entire upper body into the box; she cannot will her arm to straighten and extend into the box. Once her upper body is in the box and her right arm can reach the cranes, she focuses on capturing a crane against her palm and fingers. She tightens her fingers and sits back up with the crane. Then she tries to release her fingers so the crane falls in her lap. More often than not she gives up and takes the crane from her right hand with her left. When that happens, I take the crane, toss it back in the box, and tell her to start over. Her teachers observe the struggle with admiration and a bit of discomfort at seeing how hard Alex needs to work at everything and how hard I push her.

We hang the cranes like streamers around Alex's room—she will keep them there for years—a constant reminder of how much people care. Alex takes down an occasional crane to give to special people in her life. One of the first cranes she gives away is sent to Dr. Alden as he prepares to leave for Kenya. She sends him a brown crane because she knows that brown is his favorite color. That was one of the questions she asked during her recovery when we were so focused on reteaching her the colors. We feel so sad when it is time for Dr. Alden to leave. We have not seen him since we left Wisconsin but knowing he is a phone call or even a flight away reassures us. We keep in touch with him via email. Alex makes short videos for him and I email them for her. Alex keeps a video record of her accomplishments. Almost all of her videos begin with "Hi, Dr. Alden!" Early videos only have those three words. One video at the Ronald McDonald House in Florida says, "Hi, Dr. Alden. This is a slug." Alex wants to share things that are important to her with Dr. Alden. We haven't sent him all the videos but we think of him all the time. Our connection with Dr. Alden continues to be an important part of our lives. When Alex makes notable progress, she is often most excited about sharing it with Dr. Alden. He is her "person."

Preparing for School

Alex progresses so well that returning to school in August seems possible. Alex is determined to return to seventh grade with her friends. What classes should she take? She can't really read; we spend most of the summer reading the same book, *One Fish, Two Fish, Red Fish, Blue Fish.* It takes us almost the entire summer to finish it. Not quite seventh-grade reading material.

She can't write. Although she works on making letters pretty well with her left hand, she doesn't know what words to write. She still struggles to speak in sentences. What classes should she take in school?

I go over the dilemma with anyone willing to discuss it, which is just about everyone. I decide to enroll Alex in computers, art, and mathematics. Every minute has to count just like it does at home. I choose computers for the obvious reason that she will likely need to rely on technology for help in written communication and reading. I choose art because she loves it and I fi gure that using her left hand in art will help her write better. Math is a clear choice because, as a mathematics educator, I know I can help her make sense of the subject. She needs reading but she is so far behind that I think it will be too frustrating for her. She can barely read anything.

I ask her speech therapist to work on reading in addition to the forty-fi ve minutes or more I work with her on reading every day at home. We use reading fl ashcards every day. I make tons of them. I use words that I remember being important from my early days as an elementary school teacher. I go online and fi nd the Dolch list, a list of words that should become sight words, and make fl ashcards with them on index cards. Alex adds words as well: the days of the week and months of the year. Plus, she adds our names, including her own. It is just crazy that she needs a fl ashcard to learn to recognize her own name. I try not to focus on these things or I will go insane. Instead, I break down what I think she needs to work on and prioritize things so that we focus on things that are the most urgent, things that I know she will be successful with to maintain her motivation, and things that I know she will need much practice with to accomplish. I try to keep a mix of these three categories during my reading sessions with her.

I fi nd it interesting to see how she reads. With words like "that," she has to fi nd ways to sound them out. With words like "September," she looks at the fl ashcard, then whispers all the months of the year in order until she gets to September and then she says the word. She can recite the months in order because that is like a song and she remembers songs. Th at part of her brain is intact. With months that start with the same letter, like

"May" and "March," she uses the same strategy but often gets the two months confused. So she can read some words but not all of them. When she sees the month, she knows it is a month, she just doesn't know which month without using this additional strategy. She uses sayings she learned prior to the stroke to get to some of the words. With those words, she must have the knowledge to be able to read them someplace in her brain but she is not able to speak them without relying on other cues. Sometimes the cues mess her up. For example, whenever she tries to read the word "off" she actually says "dark." After some probing, I learn that this is because when you turn the lights off it gets dark. The way her damaged brain works fascinates me. I try to maintain an academic perspective of making sense of her brain rather than focusing on its damage. Again, it is important for my own sanity.

We use the karaoke machine we sent to Jessica for her birthday. I play songs she knows, like "The Climb," so she will sing them and see the words and form associations. The machine has two microphones and we sing together, just like we do everything else. It is fun but it doesn't help her to read. She knows the songs and doesn't bother to look at the words on the monitor. Still, we have fun singing.

We use a timer for reading activities. She tries to beat her previously held records on reading the most words she can in a minute. This motivates her. I find it surprising that she does not feel sad by the fact that she gets stuck at reading twelve words on flashcards successfully in one minute for so long. She feels motivated to improve without getting caught up in the idea of how far she has to go. I try to emulate that position. Back in Wisconsin, while Alex was sedated and I asked Dr. Alden what to expect from Alex, he had led us to believe it reasonable to expect she would maintain her vegetative state. When we tell Alex she is doing so well, that there was some thought she would be like a vegetable, she raises her chin and says, "Yeah, a cucumber!" Because we don't know her capabilities—we only know that she was supposed to be a vegetable—we don't get too caught up on it either. We just work and work. Whenever Alex shows signs of losing motivation—a rare occurrence—I remind her of the vegetable she could have been. She responds with, "I'm not a cucumber!" and she renews her effort.

Walking the Walk

Time at home consists of doing her OT exercises, PT exercises, working on mathematics, and reading. Alex's daily living activities, such as getting dressed or showered, take a good part of the day as well. The most frustrating part of the day is getting Alex to eat. It seems like we spend hours and hours on eating. She just isn't interested. I provide her with excellent choices. I make pancakes with bananas and chocolate chips, French toast from homemade bread, grilled cheese sandwiches, tuna melts, pizza from scratch, black beans and rice, every soup imaginable, chocolate cake, and apple pie. Everything tastes great—I make sure to check. It kills me. I think I gain ten pounds sitting at the table with her while she tries to eat. Apparently I am the only one doing the eating. Alex's taste buds seem different since the stroke. We have disastrous dinner times. I go all out making a sumptuous dinner and Alex pours ranch dressing, Caesar dressing, mustard, and Parmesan cheese all over whatever I make and then still won't eat it. Jessica looks at Alex's dinner plate, gags, and runs from the table. Part of Jessica's OCD involves gagging and even vomiting from things or even thoughts she finds disgusting. In second grade, her teachers had to orchestrate where Jessica sat at the lunch table so she would not end up next to boys who made messes of their lunch trays. I had warned the teachers about Jessica but it took her vomiting on the cafeteria floor before they understood the severity of her aversion to mixing food she felt did not belong together. I don't have a big enough dinner table to keep Jessica from seeing Alex's plate, so dinnertime borders on comical.

It is the end of summer and we have made significant progress. Alex is transitioning to walking with a regular cane rather than the cane with the base made of four prongs she came home with. In order to transition from the four-prong cane to a less stable cane, Alex needs to rely less on the cane. How can we get her to trust herself? I remember reading about mirror box therapy before the stroke. I don't remember where I read it or exactly what it was about, other than it had something to do with using a mirror image of your good limb to trick your brain into moving the impaired limb properly. Well, I can't figure out how to make that work with the entire half of Alex's body but I think that helping Alex to see herself walk might help. We buy a cheap full-length mirror light enough to be carried easily. Marc or I hold it in front of Alex while the other one of us stands behind her, holding onto a belt we fasten around her waist to use if she begins to fall. Alex walks toward the mirror while the person holding the mirror walks backward down the hallway, giving Alex space to keep walking. We do this over and over again, helping Alex to try to stand up tall and move her right leg forward. Lifting her leg is extremely difficult. Her foot drags.

Marc reads about a device that sends electric stimulation to the nerves responsible for lifting the foot. We try to get insurance to buy it for us because we just know it will help Alex walk. They deny it and we decide to spend the thousands of dollars for it anyway and even buy an additional device to stimulate Alex's hand. We will do anything and spare no expense to help rehabilitate Alex to her full potential. Both devices help but neither are miracle cures. There is no miracle cure, just hard work supported by anything we can find to stimulate or motivate. Certain styles and fashion statements seem to motivate Alex. Her new cane is purple with butterflies all over it. She gets a pastel blue backpack for school and has my mom embroider a big pink flamingo on it. Marc worries that it looks childish, and I suppose it does somewhat. I feel that it is another example of how happy Alex is. She feels so proud of herself and seems to enjoy life even though she works nonstop.

All the work at home is tough on Jessica. She just sits around trying to help but mostly spends her time reading. I think she reads every book in the library in this one summer. No question that we push her to the side. I don't have much choice. My parents need time to rest and renew after being at our sides and often apart from one another during the previous four months. Marc is back at work. With just the girls and me at home, Alex takes up all my time.

Marc's sister Sherri offers to take Jessica with her on vacation to North Carolina for two weeks. Earlier we had planned to send Jessica with Marc's other sister, Valerie, for a few weeks as well. However Valerie's daughter was diagnosed with severe aplastic anemia just one month ago. She was sent to a hospital in New York City far from her home in Florida by medical airplane to undergo a bone marrow transplant with her nine-year-old brother as the donor. She is only eight. She will spend over a year at the hospital in New York. Valerie and her family were actually on their way to visit Alex at the rehab hospital when her daughter's symptoms emerged. She went straight to the hospital from there. This is quite a year for our extended family.

Jessica jumps at the opportunity to go away with Sherri. I will be able to focus all my energy on working with Alex without feeling guilty about Jessica. She will have a great time. Alex and

I drive her to the prearranged meeting point so she can drive to North Carolina with Sherri and her cousins, and her puke bucket of course. Alex feels sad to have Jessica leave but she also understands why it makes sense.

After we say good-bye to Jessica and begin to drive back to Orlando, things spiral out of control once again.

24

Spasms

Alex begins spasming in the car. This happened a few times the previous week when Alex was in therapy but not as severe or for as long. I sort of ignored them. I don't know why I didn't recognize them as spasms or maybe I thought if I ignored them they would just go away. The spasms are difficult to describe. Her right hand sort of jams against her face and gets stuck there. Sometimes, often actually, she bites it when it is there. This lasts for maybe thirty seconds and then it happens again a few minutes later. It is terrifying. Are these seizures? They sure look like it. I know that brain injuries can cause seizures. Alex had a seizure while we were still in the hospital in Wisconsin but I thought that was from lowering her medication too quickly. Is it happening again? It doesn't look the same.

I call her pediatrician, Dr. Conway, on my cell phone as I drive and she says to come straight to her office and call when we get close. We are an hour away and it is a long hour. Dr. Conway meets us in the parking lot. She sees Alex spasming, brings us directly to an examining room, and calls the hospital. She suggests I try to contact Dr. Alden, the expert everyone surrounding Alex's care now turns to. I call his cell phone and though he is in surgery he manages to help us. He is completely committed to supporting us with Alex's care. He takes control and says that Alex needs to be admitted to the hospital. He contacts Dr. Patel, the neurosurgeon from Florida who had originally sent us to Wisconsin. The gears are in motion.

When we get to the hospital, we begin a twenty-four-hour video EEG to see if she is having seizures. Gluing the electrodes all over her scalp is so much easier to take this time compared to when she was in the coma with her skull out. Marc arrives at the hospital and we meet with a neurologist and Dr. Patel, who is in communication with Dr. Alden. However, neither of the doctors in Florida has ever used a DBS. Now they are in a situation that requires them to not only use a DBS for the first time, but use one on a child with a severely damaged brain. This has never been done—anywhere. It is Friday evening. We have the undivided attention of both a neurosurgeon and a neurologist brainstorming with us as we communicate with a neurosurgeon in another state. A representative from the company that makes the DBS is on her way to the hospital to help with turning it on and programming it. The support amazes me. We have a team that believes in Alex.

Coincidentally, the attending pediatric doctor is the same doctor who worked with Alex three years prior when she came in with pneumonia—the first doctor who thought Alex was feigning ill for attention. I wonder if he even remembers taking that position with Alex so long ago—assuming she was malingering. Alex's pediatrician warns me we will see him again. She also tells him a brief summary of what has happened with Alex over the last three years. As soon as I learn that he is the same doctor, I know what I will do. I show him the video of Alex spasming prior to her having brain surgery—it is crucially important to me that he sees that what he saw in Alex three years earlier was not a child feigning illness for attention. What he saw was a very difficult disease to diagnose but one that deserved more attention, more of an open mind. I think he makes this connection. He treats her much differently this time. I hope it helps him to think about his past actions as well as how he will respond to difficult cases in the future so that he will never again jump to a conclusion with other patients as he did with Alex.

The DBS

Alex is spasming every few minutes. They aren't seizures but they sure look like it. She is incapacitated again. How can this be happening? How many times have we said that over the last three years?

Marc and I discuss options with the neurologist and the neurosurgeon and, based on Dr. Alden's suggestion, we begin programming the DBS. We are glad we have the DBS as a tool to fight this, although we don't know if it will even help. There are no research reports or articles we can read to give us a sense of what to expect; there are no other cases like Alex's. We start trying medications in addition to the DBS to help give Alex relief now. Even these are being used in ways that are different from what their labels suggested. We have to do something.

Until now the DBS had been something we felt paranoid about but not something we used. The DBS ends up being something that changes the way you live. Not in major ways but it cannot be ignored, even when it isn't turned on. We are unable to use certain devices to stimulate her muscles during therapy because they might cause damage to her brain by transmitting an electrical charge through the DBS deep into her brain. It limits some of our efforts. We remember being told that Alex cannot have the strongest level of MRI and she can't have any MRIs any place but to her head. She cannot go through the regular security process at the airport. She cannot linger in a doorway of a place that has a security screening area like a library or department store. She needs to walk through those doorways in the very center. She cannot be near large magnets like those found in very large speakers at a concert. All of these constraints are because of her DBS. Certain devices, such as very strong magnets, can turn it on or off unpredictably if she gets too close to them. Basically, she has foreign objects in her body that require attention.

Before we had Alex's teeth cleaned, we had to have the dentist call the DBS manufacturer to see if the cleaning equipment was safe. As it turned out, tech support suggested the power cord not rest over her chest where the DBS battery resides.

We have to make sure that Alex's battery stays charged. As you may recall, we chose to implant a rechargeable battery because it requires replacement less frequently. Battery replacement requires surgery and we want to delay more surgery for as long as possible for obvious reasons. This means we have to remember to recharge the battery every few weeks. Placing a device over Alex's chest where the battery is in place and leaving it there for one to two hours recharges it. The trick is in getting the charger in just the right place so it syncs with the battery in Alex's chest. This is not typically a problem with Alex because she is so thin, but we've heard it can be a challenge. Alex finds the charging process uncomfortable and tries to avoid it until Marc and I remind her that her manual says that if her battery completely loses charge two times it will need to be surgically replaced. That bit of information tends to make her much more compliant. But how strange is it that Alex has a user's manual? As new parents, we beg for manuals on how to take care of our children. Be careful what you beg for. . . .

Once Alex's spasms emerge, we begin programming her DBS. The primary use for the DBS is for Parkinson's disease suff erers. With that disease, the DBS works immediately. You program it and the shaking diminishes. With spasms, it isn't so easy. It can take weeks or even months for a change to occur. The representative from the DBS manufacturer spends so much time with us explaining the process and making sure Alex understands it. Still, we feel anxious.

Between the DBS and the medication, Alex's spasms are somewhat controlled but certainly not gone. We head home with a child still spasming and so scared that she will end up right where she started. Marc and I are each a mess as well. How much more of this can we take?

We are determined to keep going. Alex is scheduled to start school in a few short weeks. She will just have to go to school with the spasms if we can't control them completely. They begin to look more like signs of Tourette's syndrome than anything else. People go to school with Tourette's and deal with the repercussions and Alex will too. We just feel so bad for her to have one more thing to deal with. It sure seems unfair.

Going Back to School

We have a series of meetings to prepare for Alex's return to school. The teachers and administrators are terrifi c. Alex will need a one-on-one aide and the administrators assign the same aide who worked with Alex before the stroke to work with her again. Th is is the best-case scenario as Alex and Miss Sue have a great relationship. Miss Sue came to see Alex at our home over the summer. She seems to be able to make sense of Alex's speech and assists her in communicating with others. Th is is probably a result of the strong bond they formed prior to the stroke. Alex likes and trusts her. We feel relieved imagining Miss Sue helping Alex to succeed in school by pushing her to achieve what she can and fi lling in the gaps as necessary. Alex, meanwhile, will work to gain knowledge about the subjects she'll be taking and will simultaneously rebuild the knowledge she lost.

Alex chooses to attend the meetings to plan her schedule and she is clearly a participant in the discussion. The guidance counselor gives Alex the schedule I request so she will only need to attend school the first three periods of the day, leaving the rest of the day for OT, PT, and speech therapy. Even with three classes, the schedule is daunting. Alex will attend school from nine a.m. till eleven thirty a.m., drive an hour to get to therapy, attend therapy for two to three hours, drive an hour to get home, eat dinner, and begin homework.

Alex is quite an interesting individual at this point. Any startling noise or flashing light causes her to spasm, smashing her right hand into her face or making loud noises. She throws anything that happens to be in her left hand when the spasm starts. The spasms typically last less than a minute but they are disruptive. She also has very little inhibition with regard to just about anything, much to Jessica's chagrin. Alex will begin dancing when she hears a song that strikes her regardless of where she is—in a restaurant, a parking lot, a waiting area for therapy. She makes everyone who is witness to these performances smile—everyone but Jessica. She loves music; she can identify a song playing as background music in a store when I'm not even aware there is music playing. Jessica doesn't mind that Alex identifies the music—she minds the dancing; Jessica feels so embarrassed when attention is drawn to Alex's dancing. When Alex begins dancing in the parking lot outside of California Pizza Kitchen, Jessica runs to the minivan, slams the door, climbs into the far backseat, and tries to make herself disappear. She is mortified. Alex doesn't care. Alex's lack of inhibition is due to her brain damage. We've been told it is something she will eventually learn to control. That would be good. . . .

One funny example of her lack of inhibition occurs at that first school-planning meeting. Alex and I are meeting with Alex's teachers, guidance counselor, and principal in a conference room. We all sit around a large table. I am always on Alex's case about her posture, aware that most stroke victims end up slouching and having bad posture due to weakened muscles. I am determined to keep this from being the case with Alex. During Alex's OT sessions at the hospital, we had begun telling her to "stick her boobies out" to get her to sit up straight. We said it so often that it eventually got shortened to "boobies out!" and I say it to her constantly. I guess that says something about my inhibitions as well; maybe Alex's issues are inherited rather than a result of the brain damage. . . . As we sit in this meeting, Alex grows bored. She looks over at her principal, a proper-looking woman who appears to be in her early forties. She is new to this school and meeting Alex for the first time, and she also happens to be slouching. Alex says in a very clear, loud voice, "Boobies out!" I think I'm going to die and Alex will be placed on hospital/homebound instruction rather than be able to attend class with the other middle school students.

The principal handles it beautifully. I quickly explain what Alex means and the principal looks her straight in the eye and says, "You're right; I am slouching" and sits up straight. I know we will be okay. This school will be great for Alex. Being in the education field, I am aware of situations where public schools don't always meet the needs of their students with special needs. That will not to be the case with this school. We are so fortunate.

It is the first day of school. Marc goes to school with Alex and helps Alex explain her situation to her classmates. It is finally time for them to truly know her story. Because Alex does not yet have the capacity to communicate well enough to tell it herself, Marc does—however, not without prior approval from Alex. I feel proud of him for this but sad that I have to work today and can't be there myself. It feels difficult to let go of the control I've taken for so long, but it is time.

Alex spasms in school—many times. It happens every time the bell rings, during a fire alarm, when students clap or drop books, with any loud, unexpected noise. The other students stare. However, they handle it well. Alex feels embarrassed, but just as she does with so many things, she just handles it. For the most part, the other students treat Alex well. I think her great attitude and the smile she always wears helps students to accept her. Students work with her in groups and even tease her in appropriate ways. One student in her computer class tries to get her to say "oink" so she will keep saying it. She still gets stuck on that word and repeats it over and over again. I don't think the boy was being mean. I think he might actually have been flirting. Alex is very cute. We don't know the boy's name because Alex still doesn't remember anyone's name at school. She has hers down now but not her teachers' or even her best friends' names.

Alex eats lunch at school once per week. When she feels she can handle the noise with her spasms, she sits with her old group of friends. Even though she can't remember their names, they accept her. She is unable to participate in the types of conversations that go on in the lunchroom but her friends find ways to include her just the same. They talk to her about boys and other things you might expect from seventh-grade girls and Alex mostly listens. School is still tough but it could have been so much worse.

We have a childcare provider now. My mother and Alex met her at the hospital during therapy where she volunteers. Michelle is terrific. She is a senior at the university where I work, majoring in health sciences. She plans to graduate in May and go on to graduate school to become an occupational therapist. What a find!

Michelle picks Alex up from school several times per week while I work. She brings her to her therapies and takes notes for Marc and me so we can support the therapists' efforts at home. When she picks Alex up from school on days that Alex feels upset, she can turn Alex's mood around by the time Alex gets to therapy so that Alex will get the most out of it. Michelle is twenty years old and sort of a cool big sister to Alex. She even gets Alex to enjoy hip-hop, something she would certainly not have learned from me. Although I must admit that I listen to it now too. I guess Michelle influences us all.

Michelle does so much to keep Alex's spirits high, but we also feel we need the support of Alex's psychologist, the surfer from Cocoa Beach. He was instrumental in Alex's "Yes I Can" attitude before her stroke. He also helped me to know whether my parenting was appropriate. I am living on gut feelings now. None of what I am figuring out was in *What to Expect When You're Expecting* or *What to Expect the First Year*. I am reraising my daughter by the seat of my pants. The first time around, I read both books from cover to cover and did everything they said. They didn't have any chapters on what to expect when your twelve-year-old daughter has a stroke and you have to start all over again because she wants to regain everything she lost immediately and you want that for her too. I have no idea how hard to push Alex, and I push her pretty hard. I need Dr. Stewart for reassurance.

Dr. Stewart

We set up appointments for both girls in Cocoa Beach. They see Dr. Stewart for an hour each. What we do with the hour they each need to wait is just brilliant. Dr. Stewart's wife is an artist. Sherri paints the most beautiful sea life on canvas. Her art is whimsical and relaxing yet simultaneously deep, if that is possible. Many of her paintings include sayings that can be related both to life's struggles and its rewards. She is tall and gorgeous with long blond hair. She dresses like an artist and has a very easy way about her. Her studio is right next door to Dr. Stewart's office overlooking the ocean. Her art is all over the walls; some of it is actually painted on the walls. There are blank canvases and paintbrushes in all sizes to choose from and every color of paint. The girls are free to choose what they want to paint, what colors they want to use, and on what size canvas.

I arrange for one daughter to meet with Dr. Stewart while the other daughter has a private art lesson with Sherri. Then they switch. Jessica paints ocean scenes, palm trees, peace signs, and owls. Alex paints kissing fish, mermaids, pelicans, and giraffes. Jessica spends weeks and weeks on each piece of work. Alex finishes one after another during her sessions. Both the psychology appointments and the art lessons turn out to be excellent therapy.

Dr. Stewart helps Alex see that she is a miracle while simultaneously calling her out when necessary. He gives me the courage to keep pushing her and to accept no less from her than I feel she is able to give. He reassures me that I should continue to go with my instincts. He meets with Marc and me on occasion to help us maintain a shared vision of our expectations for Alex and how we might support her in meeting them. He also helps us to begin to understand Jessica's struggles.

Jessica is hurting. She feels nobody even sees her anymore. They only see Alex. She is right in so many ways. I feel terrible for her. Alex is such a miracle and changes so quickly that everyone wants to talk about her, see her, and tell us how great she is doing. Jessica is left in the background. Some people still ask about Jessica, but not many.

I begin taking a much closer look at the situation and I don't like what I see. Th is is taking its toll on Jessica. I begin a concerted eff ort to spend more time with Jessica and to make sure that people interact with her as well. How people treat her isn't on purpose, but it isn't acceptable either. Jessica still struggles with this. Writing this book doesn't help. She is an amazing child. She knows that writing this book will bring even more attention to Alex but she says to do it anyway. She even off ers to contribute several chapters. She says that people need to know Alex's story. She will handle whatever comes from it and she will go one step further. She will contribute to the project by sharing her story in her own words, as painful as it feels.

GETTING MY LIFE BACK (BY JESSICA DIXON)

I'm known in my family to get easily embarrassed, scared, and stressed. It has been going on for years. When I was three I ran out of a theater while watching *A Bug's Life* because I was terrifi ed of bugs and the fat ladybug was coming for me. When I was six I ran out of the movie *Cars* because an "embarrassing" scene came on. After several times of my parents dashing out of the theater to catch me, a minute too late, I was forced to sit between them to stop my fl eeing. As you might guess, Alex's lack of a fi lter kills me. I am quite shy unless you know me, and her moments of random dancing and singing activate my fi ght-or-flight response. Next thing I know, I am hiding in a car. Alex's moments of stardom are like fl ash mobs with one participant, unless my mom joins in. My dad at least doesn't start in on the performance, but has learned from experience to solemnly stand there until the onslaught ends. I busy myself with hiding or pretending I don't know her.

Another issue is my "motor mouth." I am meek and little around strangers, but when I am comfortable I am still little but more like a hyperactive chipmunk. My friends think I'm insane and I talk a mile per minute. This can cause complications at home. Mostly Alex sits there in a daze after getting lost the moment my mouth opens. This greatly irritates everyone and I am constantly nagged to slow down. I think my parents use Alex as an excuse to have me slow down so they can understand me as well. I "attempt" to pause "often" to give her time to speak, but apparently I don't do it enough. This mostly results in Alex getting frustrated with me and not believing I am trying to help. Old habits die hard.

I started tennis lessons. Everyone has their thing that they do and mine is school. It is fun to branch away from the usual. Also, tennis is something that doesn't involve Alex. I don't have to slow down or stand there awkwardly while people discuss my sister. I am finally getting my life back. I feel this way more when I am doing things that don't involve Alex. I'm hoping that soon I will feel this way with Alex as well.

· ·

25

Straight A's

Alex successfully completes the fi rst half of the school year and even manages to maintain straight A's on her report card. Her aide reads tests for her and records for Alex as well. Alex has unlimited time to take tests and she uses it. The school provides everything in their power to help her succeed and she responds with amazing motivation.

Alex basically starts over with math. I use only the best teaching practices to help her make sense of mathematics. Her math teacher at school is a colleague of mine. You can't get any better. Alex says, "A stroke and a coma and now I like math." I feel good about that until I remember I was her mother the fi rst time she learned math as well. I hadn't been as helpful in ensuring she understood the mathematics so she could like it when she was younger.

This time I don't teach her how to perform a procedure like adding fractions without ensuring she understands the concept fi rst. We discuss contexts like putting leftover pizza pieces from diff erent pizzas together in a box to determine how much of a pizza we have in all. We draw pictures to represent slices of pizza and how we can determine how much we have all together if one pizza is cut in eighths and the other sixteenths. We do all this before even writing a fraction symbol. At school, her teacher uses inquiry methods with her students; she expects students to make claims about mathematics and then back those claims with explanations and justifications. Alex is no exception. Unlike most of her other classes, in math class the students sit in groups and discuss the mathematics problems before discussing them with the entire class. Alex participates. She says it is the one class where students begin to know her again and accept her. She participates in class discussions by using numbers, words, drawings, gestures, and classmates to help make her point. When she writes a seven but calls it a six her group mates just correct her and move on without making an issue out of it. Her teacher holds her accountable to high expectations. She wishes all her classes provided ways for her to participate and become one of the group as this one does. When Dr. Stephan, her math teacher, leaves the school to take a university position in another state, Alex gives her one of the paper cranes. This teacher's belief in Alex is clearly meaningful.

We are resolute regarding the types of experiences to which we expose Alex in the classes she selects, the ways she studies, and even in the vacations we take. We think about every choice we make. Dr. Stewart encourages us to stimulate her brain in many different ways. I think it makes a difference. Over the winter break, we plan to go to Washington, DC, to visit the Smithsonian. We hope this will help her to prepare for the geography class she will begin taking at midyear.

The trip is great. It snows and she is captivated—so many things have the power to captivate her. She wants us to take pictures of everything in the Smithsonian, with the caveat that she has to be in every picture. She takes pictures with statues of Elvis posing with a facial expression just like his. There is actually an eerie resemblance in some of the pictures. She takes

pictures with jeweled pianos, airplanes, and rockets—wanting
to know about everything—seemingly hearing about things
she had once known for the fi rst time. Each night she returns
to the hotel room and writes in a journal. She is adamant about
recording every aspect of her life. Each entry takes at least an
hour to write but she perseveres.

December 29, 2010

Lincoln Memorial

The Lincoln Memorial was beautiful. It made me feel
patriotic and spiritual. From the top of the stairs I saw the
Washington Monument. The water was pretty and the
monument was tall.

—*Alex*

She is adamant about many things. If she gets something
in her mind, she doesn't let it go—like meeting the president,
for example. So proud of her accomplishments, she is sure the
president will want to meet her. We tell her how unlikely that
is, but to her, anything is possible. She talks about it constantly
and looks for him everywhere. We fi nally have a picture of her
taken at a kiosk where the president is later photoshopped into
the image to look like he is shaking hands with her. I never would
have paid fi ve dollars for something so ridiculous prior to Alex's
stroke, but in our new life I am less likely to say no without
thinking. Now I pause and think that it's only fi ve dollars and it
will make her so happy. It does. She shows everyone her picture
with the president and I am surprised by how many people are
fooled. I guess Alex isn't the only one who believes she is worthy
of meeting him. The picture will satisfy her until she meets the
president for real and I don't doubt she will. Anything is possible

with Alex. Experiences like this remind me of the saying that children with special needs are gifts. It takes having a child with special needs to realize this. She requires more work on my part and clearly more stress, but I feel so fortunate to just be in her presence, to learn from her unique perspective that feeling like you met the president can be almost as good as meeting him.

Alex seems to bloom in every aspect of her being. All of her efforts toward recovery seem to cause even more areas of her brain to be stimulated. She walks better, eventually switching to a foldable cane so she can leave it in her backpack for parts of the day and walk without one. She talks better, finding more and more words and making her point without assistance much more often. She writes better. It doesn't take long for her penmanship to surpass mine, even writing with her left hand. She certainly reads better than she had during the summer.

We spent the entire summer reading one Dr. Seuss book and by January she was reading Magic Tree House books in a matter of weeks. We move well beyond reading flashcards.

At midyear she completes her art and computer classes. It is time to pick new classes. Alex chooses to continue with math and adds science and geography to her schedule. She also adds reading through hospital/homebound instruction. This is a much more rigorous schedule. We all worry she might not be able to keep up.

Motivated to maintain straight A's and fully recover, Alex works nonstop. She memorizes states and capitals and can locate them on maps. She has me read her geography and science book chapters to her over and over again until she can make sense of the content. I make index cards with study questions and she practices them with her father, her sister, her grandparents, her caregiver, her aide, and me. I write the question on one side of the card and the answer on the other. I make two sets of identical cards so she can self-check or whoever is testing her can check for accuracy. I do this because Alex needs to both see and hear the contents of both sides of the cards. She practices by matching the prompts with the answers as she looks at them while someone reads their content. I begin by giving her two options; I put two different prompts with their answers face up on the table for her to place in pairs. When she gets those correct, I add another pair and mix up all three for her to match. I add another when she gets those correct. It is a slow process. We continue until she has one group of the entire set of cards. Repetition is important, but still, her memory is impressive. With cards that are difficult for her to remember, I make up silly sayings to help her. For example, to remember that the capital of Colorado is Denver, I say and sing to her in a silly voice, "John Denver sang, rocky mountain high, Colorado." She laughs at me but she also remembers. She is unstoppable. There are times when teachers who didn't know Alex before the stroke email me and say that I am pushing her too hard, that she needs more rest. It almost feels as though they think I am pushing to the point of being abusive. I am glad to have Dr. Stewart for reassurance. I trust him and so does Alex. Whenever I meet with him, my eyes linger on the paper crane displayed prominently on his bookshelf. Alex does not give those out lightly, further proof of her trust. The teachers don't understand that Alex is pushing herself. I push her to be motivated and provide opportunities to learn and recover and she does the rest.

Odyssey of the Mind

Alex wants to rejoin her Odyssey of the Mind team. How will this work? Odyssey of the Mind involves problem solving and spontaneous responses. Can she possibly be a contributing member of a team? Nobody really knows.

Ms. Poarch, her Odyssey of the Mind coach from the year before, the one who had been involved with the thousand paper cranes, says we should give it a try. She pulls Alex's team together and tells them about Alex's desire to rejoin the team. She tells them that it is their choice and they will need to vote to decide if they will support Alex as a member. The vote is unanimous. The team wants Alex back.

Alex becomes the main character in the skit the team writes and performs as part of their competition. They work on it for months. Alex is not able to help much with building the set but she is creative and helps in many ways. Alex even comes up with the idea for the project. The task for this year is to make a Rube Goldberg machine, a contraption that replaces a simple machine with something complicated, purposefully over-engineered. The team spends weeks searching for a simple device they can use as the basis of their machine. Alex tears apart our kitchen examining appliances and utensils looking for the perfect idea. It is important to her to contribute the idea for the device because she knows there are other aspects of the project with which she will not be much help, such as building the set for the skit. Th is is another instance where she is single-minded about something. She is beginning to drive me crazy. She talks about fi nding the perfect item constantly. After one psychology session, she begs me to stop at a dollar store to peruse the aisles for ideas. I think it is just an excuse for her to shop, her new favorite pastime, but I capitulate as a result of her persistence. She fi nds a funnel in the store and knows it will be the device. She convinces her team members and takes the part in the skit of the mad scientist who designs the U.L.T., the Ultimate Liquid Transporter. The team accepts her and focuses on her strengths rather than her weaknesses. I am so proud of the group. Her team makes it to the state-level competition. Th is means so much to Alex. Ms.

Poarch's role in this opportunity is not lost on Alex; she too has one of Alex's cranes.

Toward the end of the school year, Alex receives two awards at the awards assembly—one with her Odyssey of the Mind team and another for maintaining straight A's the entire year. The previous year she had not been able to go up on the stage to get her awards. This year, there is still no ramp. However, Alex walks from where she is seated with the other students to the stage and straight up the steps! She doesn't even use a cane. Her teachers and administrators rush over to her to offer assistance in getting up the stairs. She won't take it. She walks up herself. I feel sobs of relief well up inside me and slip out. I just cry where I sit on the bleachers in the audience. I feel so proud of her and of how far she has come in just one year. I know she is proud of herself as well, but still she knows she has not come this far without help. I know for a fact that she has the smallest of her paper cranes tucked in her pocket, as she always does for important events. After the awards assembly, Alex tells me she was so excited she almost peed her pants.

I see Alex as a child—a young adult actually—determined to take her life back, determined to succeed in school and determined to succeed in life.

Focusing on the Positive

Alex does everything she can to improve. She still spasms, which embarrasses her and disrupts all around her. At first it seems that having her eat sugar stops the spasms. During a bout of spasms, we give her something sugary to eat and it seems to help. Now she is eating way too much sugar. It seems wrong. If her spasms are caused by an inappropriate response from her autonomic nervous system, as is suspected, how can dumping sugar into her be good? She spasms so much and we feel desperate. I decide to try eliminating sugar from her diet—not completely, as I don't eliminate fruit, but I decide that she will not eat anything with more than five grams of sugar per serving. I'm just guessing here but it's the best idea I have at this point so I go with it. She agrees to try. It works! In three months' time, she is basically spasm-free—spasm-free and off all medication shortly after! I don't know if it is the sugar or coincidental timing with when the DBS finally works but it really doesn't matter. Alex doesn't dwell on this significant change to her diet. She focuses on the positive.

She tries to do the same thing with her eyesight but it has yet to have the same result. After the stroke she could no longer see to the right in either eye. Think of the silly eye test where the eye doctor holds up fingers at different places in your field of vision and asks you to tell how many fingers you see. I never understood why I had to do that test. It seemed ridiculously easy. I can see how many fingers even without my contact lenses in! I now have an appreciation for the purpose of that test. Alex does not even know the fingers are there when held from anywhere beyond straight in front of her nose to her right with either eye or both eyes open. I had no idea. You just wouldn't know it with the way she interacts with her surroundings. She has accommodated for that disability so well.

Without that field of vision, she will most likely be unable to drive, which is hard news for her to take. She has always wanted to drive. The eye doctor says that it will not be possible with her vision the way it is. We found that out at the beginning of the school year. Alex was devastated. But now she is saying her vision is coming back. She says that every month she can see a little more. We feel so excited! She will be able to drive after all.

We go back to the eye doctor and the news isn't good. Her vision hasn't changed. It won't change. That part of her brain will not repair. She is devastated all over again. I ask Alex, "Why did you say you could see better if it wasn't true? I know you aren't a liar." She says she hoped that, if she believed she could see better, it would help her to see better. I tell her to keep that attitude and that science might catch up with her some day. She says she will try but in the meantime she wants a cute limo driver to drive her around. That's the spirit.

She takes a similar perspective on her state tests in school. Alex has to take state math and reading tests. These are rigorous tests. They weren't always rigorous to Alex; she had always received top scores before her stroke. I don't think she is ready to pass them but she is determined to work toward a regular high school diploma so she has to take them. The tests are administered over four days with each part of the test designed to take about an hour per day. She has extended time. She spends between fi ve to six hours on each part. A score of three is passing and the top score one can achieve is a fi ve. Her goal is to do well enough to get a score of one rather than having a test that cannot be scored because there are not enough correct answers. She takes the tests with an aide reading the math questions to her. The reading test cannot be read to her. She comes out of the testing room at the end of each day with a big smile on her face after working all day and says, "I think I got a one. I think I did it!" She knows a one is a failing score but she still feels proud of her accomplishment. I don't know of anyone else in this world that can take such a difficult situation and make it so positive.

Her eff orts pay off. She gets a two on her reading test. She actually passes her math test! She did it with half a brain. As a mathematics educator, I prepare mathematics teachers. I am often asked what to do about students with special needs because people believe they cannot succeed in math. I never used to accept this but I'm not sure I fought back with enough conviction. I would say, "All students can learn," and "You need to differentiate instruction to meet the needs of your students and they will succeed." I don't think I really had a clue regarding what was involved with truly reaching all students, or what it really means to differentiate instruction. Differentiated instruction means that students are provided with different ways of learning. What is missing is the idea that you need to determine what those ways are for individual students. I needed to figure out, along with Alex, how to help her learn. Alex has made me such a better teacher because of how she refuses to give up and because of how we have to work together to find ways to help her learn within her disability rather than by ignoring it—or worse, using it as an excuse to not learn. Her attitude—a productive disposition—has so much to do with her success.

She isn't satisfied with her reading score or with her slow reading pace. She chooses to attend reading and speech camps throughout the summer to focus on improving her reading. While other children saunter off to adventure camps or relax, Alex attends two academic camps for four hours each day, then on to PT, OT, and speech therapy. She spends the first part of the morning with graduate students at my university working with struggling readers. She reads elementary school-level books and spends weeks and weeks just trying to get through one. Her childcare provider or I pick her up from that camp and drive her across campus to the next camp. At that camp she works with graduate students in speech and communicative disorders. They help her with conversations and writing for two hours. University faculty advise the graduate students in both camps. They are drawn in to Alex's case immediately. We have long discussions about Alex's goals and how best to meet them. Both camps assign homework that we work on together at home. Nonstop work. From the second camp, she hops in the car and drives across town to the rehab facility that off ers PT, OT, and speech therapy. She attends those for two to three hours. Th is involves stretching, exercises, trying to use her right hand, and trying to walk on planks and treadmills. Sometimes her therapists give her tasks to do, such as making a peanut butter and jelly sandwich. It seems simple but it takes Alex thirty minutes and she wears more peanut butter and jelly than the sandwich does. Sometimes she has to try to put pegs in a pegboard, only to be told to take them out again. Most of the time she does things without complaining but sometimes her frustration fl ares. She says, "Th is is stupid. I'm done!" This usually occurs when she is not experiencing success with her task. These outbursts are short-lived. My response is almost always, "Are you? Just say the word and therapy will stop." At these times I feel panicked on the inside but I try to keep a tough exterior. I think she relies on it. She says, "No, let's keep going . . . ." And she returns to the task that temporarily got the best of her. Probably her least favorite task is in speech therapy, where she walks the halls outside the therapy office with the therapist reading her uninteresting passages and then asking Alex to recall details and answer questions from the passage just read. Alex struggles to do these two things at once—listen and walk. I follow along saying the responses in my mind. They are so easy but Alex gets most of them wrong. These are the times I want to say, "Th is is stupid. I'm done!" But I have nobody to say it to and nobody to call my bluff , so I keep it in and keep on going.

It isn't all work and no play. Alex also plays. She continues to use theme songs to help motivate and defi ne her. Earlier she had focused on "Lean on Me" and "The Climb." Her new theme song is "Live Like You're Dying." She wants to experience everything.

26

Living Like She's Dying

Alex lives like she's dying but everyone else lives to support Alex. Jessica continues on the sidelines so often. We try hard to include her and focus on her but we are pushed to our limits with helping Alex recover. Jessica has decided to attend sleep-away camp in North Carolina this summer. She needs a break from our family and from being around all the focus on Alex.

She chooses a traditional girls camp and to go on her own rather than with friends. She says she wants to find herself, which seems strange for an eleven-year-old. In so many ways she is wise beyond her years. She will spend three weeks at camp in North Carolina. I will drive her to North Carolina as soon as school is over.

Alex and I decide to make a road trip out of it. We drive Jessica to camp and then spend a week traveling around North Carolina and Georgia before driving back home.

Alex plans the agenda. She wants to visit Marc's mother and stepfather in North Carolina. Once there she wants to go gem mining and whitewater rafting. Following these excursions, she wants to visit Marc's father and stepmother in Georgia and go to an arcade gallery. These are all activities she had done prior to her illness. I feel that Alex feels the need to recreate her childhood and prove to herself that she can still live in it. I am worried she will be disappointed but I decide to not dissuade her and to see how things go.

We find a whitewater rafting trip with low to moderate rapids and go for it. It is fantastic! Who would have thought just a year ago that Alex would be whitewater rafting? She plays it up big. There are parts of the trip she can't do. For example, the part where you climb out of the raft and up a cliff to jump into the freezing water fifteen feet below. "Mom, please do it for me since I can't do it myself. I'll take pictures!" Her big brown eyes implore me to climb that cliff. I feel the tug much less clearly when I get to the top and am looking down into the fast-paced, cold river. Now it is too late and I have to jump. "Slap!" Entry into the water is not ideal. I have a bruise along the entire side of my thigh that lasts for weeks. I also have to endure Alex laughing about my "butt-flop" for days. But I suppose it is worth it. Farther down the river I dunk Alex off the side of the raft into the cold water in sweet revenge.

The song she lives by mentions climbing the Rocky Mountains and skydiving as well. She decides to substitute a rock-climbing wall at an arcade gallery for the Rocky Mountains and I am thrilled. We find a place in Georgia. The young man working the wall is super. He helps Alex get a few feet up the wall. I'm not sure what Alex likes better—the climbing or the cute boy helping her. Actually, I know she likes the cute boy best but I am not ready to focus on that. After he helps her climb, her name for him is "butt guy," a description of the body part he grabs on her to hoist her up the wall. I am not at all pleased with how he manages to help her climb.

During the road trip, she finds a T-shirt that says I CAN SEE CLEARLY NOW THE BRAIN IS GONE. She buys it and wears it with pride. She is proud of herself and she has every right to be. In many regards, she is happier and more outgoing than she was before she got sick so long ago. Alex hasn't gone skydiving yet but I don't doubt that she will.

Marc and I remember the day Alex was in surgery to get her skull replaced like it was yesterday. So many of our memories of this journey remain extremely vivid. On this day, we are in the waiting room during surgery and there are computers available to look at the Internet. Marc looks up sites on stroke rehabilitation and they are grim. Recovery will be slow and tenuous at best for a major stroke. Little recovery can be expected beyond the one-year mark poststroke. These websites were awful to read and contained little hope. I'm glad we stopped reading them and charted our own course filled with hope. Alex's recovery continues.

Another year has passed and she has already relearned to swim. She carried her own backpack to school all year, ate her lunch at school each day with her friends and without her aide, and even did some of her homework and schoolwork on her own. She graduated from eighth grade, is preparing for high school, and plans to earn a regular high school diploma. She makes her own bed, sets the table, helps to make her lunch, and gets herself ready for school on her own. She is becoming so independent. She still has a long way to go. She walks without a cane but she does not have a normal gait. Her right hand moves some but is not very helpful to her.

Alex has trouble keeping up with conversations and is working hard to learn how to converse with teenagers. I tell her that talking with teenagers is a mystery to many of us. She is beginning to notice that she does not keep up with her peers. She wants to read and write as fast as her friends. She wants to be completely independent. She does not see herself as disabled and will not tolerate others having that view. She went snorkeling with sharks on her eighth-grade field trip. She even went to sleep-away camp at Sea World on her own for five days. She has gone horseback riding, kayaking, and sailing. She is determined to succeed. She says she wants to be a doctor so she can help people. She wants to help people who have gone through difficulties like she has. She wants to give them a second chance at life.

Reborn

Alex continues to persevere. In Alex's school system, there is an award for students who have overcome barriers. It is called the Phoenix Award. One student is chosen from the elementary-school level, one from the middle-school level, and one from the high-school level. Alex's principal nominated Alex at the end of her eighth-grade year, her last year in middle school. This is what we submitted:

Phoenix Award Letter for Alex Dixon

Alex Dixon contracted pneumonia halfway through fourth grade. Prior to that time she was a bright, kind, and sometimes socially awkward child. She loved animals, playing the piano, art, and playing outside. The pneumonia triggered a glitch in her central nervous system and she would never fully recover from her illness. The glitch caused her body to contort and she experienced considerable pain. She missed a great deal of school and spent much of her days in hospitals seeking a cure for her illness. By the time she began sixth grade, she was confined to a wheelchair and still in pain.

Alex began sixth grade in the gifted program. She continued to excel academically as well as with art and piano. However, her condition took a significant turn for the worse halfway through sixth grade, two years after the initial onset. Her body began contorting in terrible ways, causing hundreds of dislocations every day. It seemed that she would not survive. She was flown to a hospital in the Midwest and placed in a coma in an attempt to buy time as new medications were introduced, but to no avail. On February 23, 2010, Alex underwent brain surgery as a last effort to save her life. It was her sister's tenth birthday and Alex was just twelve years old. The surgery did not go well, although it did resolve her original problems. An accident caused a massive stroke to the left hemisphere of Alex's brain. She was placed in a coma for many weeks in order to increase her likelihood of survival. Her classmates were behind her and folded a thousand paper cranes so that she might get her wish to live.

Alex survived. She came out of the coma and slowly recovered memories of her life experiences but not of her academics. She knew her family but not their names. She didn't even know her own name. She came home from the hospital in June and was determined to enter seventh grade with her peers in August. It has been just a little more than two years since her stroke. She has spent that time relearning to eat, walk, care for herself, speak, read, write, and do math. She has more determination than can be imagined. She is in regular classes with a one-on-one aide. She works nonstop. While her right hand no longer works, she is writing better than many with her left hand. She is determined to relearn piano one-handed and her artwork is beautiful. She even discarded, first the wheelchair and, eventually, her cane.

At the end of her seventh-grade year, Alex passed her state math test. She scored a level two out of five in reading. This year, she will likely pass that as well. She is an A student in regular classes. She is liked by her peers and adored by her teachers. She has a "Yes I Can" attitude that is nothing less than contagious. Alex has certainly encountered roadblocks and hardship resulting in significant disabilities over the past four years. However, her resilience, strength, and determination are unmatched and her future is wide open.

The Phoenix is said to be reborn from its own ashes to live again. Alex has been reborn to live again as well. She is bright, but in a different way than before. She is kind to all she encounters, and she is now anything but socially awkward. She is a survivor who will make the most of life.

Alex won the award. I know that everyone has obstacles but, at least to me, Alex's seem so very significant and her victories absolutely profound. She is a remarkable individual conquering adversity and thriving in who she has become while simultaneously working to become even more. She is a phoenix.

Going through Hell

Alex says my theme song is "If You're Going through Hell." The song says to keep on going right through to the other side. I believe we've done that. I don't think Alex has a sense of just how outstanding she is and how amazing her accomplishments truly are.

"Mom, I want to be good at something. I'm not good at anything. Jessica is good at reading and science. You're good at math. I'm not good at anything."

"What do you mean, Alex? You're so good at getting well."

"That's not what I mean."

"Let me think . . . . Alex, what you're good at—really good at—is giving people hope. When people spend time with you, they feel good. They feel hopeful. Your story that started with such difficulty has become such a story of hope, because of who you are and how you've chosen to handle what your life brought you."

"I guess you're right. I'm good at making people feel good. You're good at making people work hard. I'm glad you made me work hard. I love you."

Alex's story is truly something. It has such difficult beginnings, such unbelievable struggles, and such a hopeful future. Alex was given a second chance at life. I am grateful for that. I am even more grateful that she had the courage to take it.

PART VI:
PERSPECTIVES

27

Looking Back on the Journey

Alex's journey was nothing we asked for and certainly not what we intended. Her stroke was an accident during surgery, a terrible accident. However, we will never know if it also saved her life. This helps us live our lives without resentment. I can't imagine going through what we have gone through while feeling there was someone to blame. We do not harbor those feelings and we remain thankful for that and so many other things. We were losing Alex. We were losing our amazing, thoughtful, intelligent, beautiful, caring daughter. We all knew it. Then she had a stroke during surgery. It took so much from her. However, it also might have saved her. Following the stroke, her dislocations stopped, her RSD pain resolved, her foot no longer contorted, and her attitude improved. It was a stroke of luck and it gave Alex a second chance at life. She chose to take it and live her life better than anyone could have imagined. She didn't do it alone. She had a village to support her.

Writing this book helped Alex's healing process. There are parts of her journey that she did not know about, such as what occurred when she was in the coma. I read those parts of the book to her and she is able to put together a puzzle that is otherwise incomplete. She laughs when she hears about Marc holding his hands up in the air in the ICU when she had C. diff. She cries when I read the parts where doctors did not believe in her, but mostly when her own family's faith in her waivered. This is all part of her coping process as well as that of our entire family. There are many days when I sit between Alex and Jessica on the couch and read for hours. Marc can only read small portions of the manuscript at a time and he is brought to tears with every sitting. When I send the manuscript to my mother to read, she stays up all night, unable to turn away but sobbing deeply while trying to read through her tears.

I began writing *A Stroke of Luck* in earnest toward the end of Alex's first year back at school. I wrote the first draft throughout the summer following her first year back at school after the stroke and I completed the final draft during the second summer. I know that my writing the book causes Alex some growing pains and I'm sorry for that; but she knows probably more than anyone that you often have to endure pain to improve. It actually causes everyone involved to relive some terrible moments in our lives. However, I also feel it allows us to reflect on how motivation, effort, persistence, love, and positive thinking can move mountains. I like to think that the tears this book causes are balanced by the amount of hope it provides.

So many people had an effect on—and are affected by—Alex's journey. Their points of view, by definition, differ from my own. I never stopped to consider this until writing Alex's book. I asked many people to read what I had written along the way to be sure I depicted Alex's story as accurately as possible and the input was, at times, surprising. I found that I had never thought of certain events in the same way as others close to Alex had viewed them. It becomes obvious that their perspectives are crucial to an accurate view of this journey. I ask those I feel are most intricately involved in Alex's entire journey to write what strikes them, giving no other direction. The perspectives of Jessica, Marc, and my parents are included here. I am forever grateful to those who believe in Alex and support her journey. These perspectives represent a very small subset of that village.

JESSICA'S POINT OF VIEW

At first I was devastated. I rode on a plane for four hours happy as can be. I was going to see my mom, dad, and sister! We were going to talk, laugh, and hug! I especially couldn't wait to hug. By that time I was yelling at my parents on Skype because of the hurt of abandonment. At that time I thought they could have come home to see me and then fly back to Alex. I told them more than once you can't hug on Skype. When I got to the airport, instead of wearing smiles, we were all crying after talking with mom and dad face to face for five minutes. I was now a big sister and sure I would never be happy again.

Now things are looking better. Alex has become a miracle, my miracle. Now, as my sister has gotten over the big bumps of her stroke, this new life is my family's new normal. As soon as I accepted Alex the way she is and stopped comparing my sister to someone I call "old Alex," I started to be less haunted by it. Now it feels like Alex was always this way. Now I look upon the stroke curiously. How did this work? Why would that happen? Those questions are basically how I view the stroke. I am sad and happy this happened. The stroke either saved her life or made it one million times harder. How

I think of it, for my own sanity, is that it saved Alex. At first I felt bad that I had taken an interest in the thing that had hurt Alex so badly. I told Mom and she said I was healing. What was so wrong in finding out why my sister is a miracle?

Then I started to feel jealous and hurt. I was hurt during the early stroke rehabilitation but I didn't feel hurt because of what was happening to me, I was only hurting for my sister. I didn't feel jealous at all. Now after the stroke, it's finally safe enough to let out all the feelings I held inside me during the sickness and the stroke. These are feelings I didn't even know I felt, or the ones that I did know I felt but I didn't know I felt them so strongly. For example, most people talk to Alex, most people want to see Alex. Many of our family friends, my parents' friends, and my parents' coworkers don't realize that the stroke affects the whole family. I am very grateful for the people who realize the effect it has had on me. People reading this book are reading about Alex, so they wouldn't know the bad things that happened to me around the time of the stroke and so I will write them now. I was without my mom and dad first for three weeks, then for five weeks. My dad came home, but not my mom. I thought my family would only be gone two days. I asked every day I saw my mom and dad on Skype, before my birthday and before I knew what was happening, if they would make it home for my birthday. Every time they said they would, then later on they'd say "probably," and guess what, I spent my birthday without my grandpa, my mom, my dad, and Alex. It was just my grandma and me. They didn't make it. At the time I didn't know why and now I feel guilty for being angry with them. It is like I can't win.

I want adults who know Alex and are with her and me to include me in conversations and actually listen to what I say. To listen to me like the way most people listen to Alex. I don't want pity; people get nothing done by sitting around feeling sorry for themselves. I want to change the way people act. I want people around the world in the shadow of their injured siblings to have people include them. If you know someone with an injured sibling or a sibling fighting an illness, they are probably in their sibling's shadow. So when you see them, include the uninjured or well brother or sister in conversations.

I am not mad at Alex. I know that she has it worse than me and I know it isn't her fault. I'm not mad at my mom, grandma, or grandpa. I'm sometimes mad at my dad. I deserve to be mad those times but the reason he treats me unfairly is because he doesn't know how to treat Alex. Even so, it still hurts, but I couldn't have asked for a better dad. I've got the kindest, most understanding, and sweetest family in the world.

Grandma's Point of View

While speaking to relatives and friends, the first question I hear from them is, "How is Alex doing?" My reply: "She's a miracle child." One only has to reflect on this ordeal to understand my response. The change was a life-altering event for Alex as well as for our whole extended family. My role changed from doting grandma and mother to a wonderful family to caregiver, supporter, and worrier.

What began as a few days of childcare for Jessica became a nine-week emotional roller coaster for the entire family. I assumed the responsibility of mother and father in addition to my role as grandmother to a child who dearly missed her family. So we tried to cope, Jessica and I, although life was difficult. Every night she would Skype with her parents, after which I held her in my arms as she cried until sleep took over. I devoted myself to providing a stable and safe environment for Jessica—play dates, sleepovers, dinners out, and visits from family and friends provided some diversion for both of us.

I managed my life by volunteering at Jessica's school every day as a tutor to children experiencing academic difficulties. It felt natural to be back in a classroom setting because I had been a teacher for nearly thirty years before retiring. This enabled me to push the realities from the forefront of my mind and provided me with a release from the stresses in my life. I returned to my home every few weeks to pick up mail and connect with a few friends who were my immediate support group during these difficult times. I also lived with my cell phone in my side pocket, using it as a constant connection to my daughter Marni, my husband, and close relatives as a means of maintaining a modicum of hope and reassurance.

After many weeks—and once Juli and Alex transitioned to the rehab hospital in Florida—Marc had to return to work. I replaced him at Alex's side. We were a new team: Harvey, Juli, Alex, Jessica to some extent, and I. We gathered all of our professional and life experiences to embark on a path to facilitate Alex's rehabilitation. The hospital staff was amazed and impressed with the impact we had in accelerating her progress. We played games, read to her, sang songs, encouraged verbal interaction, and, most of all, believed in her ability to successfully recover.

As Alex continues to progress, I am able to resume my role as a doting grandmother to both Alex and Jessica. We talk, we laugh, we cook together, do crafts, shop for clothes, go to museums, and, most of all, enjoy each other's company.

Grandpa's Point of View

The telephone call from my daughter that started this journey in earnest for me was startling. Juli, who is fiercely independent and almost never asks for assistance, suggested I catch the next available flight to Wisconsin to assist in keeping Alex "safe." I had no sense of what this meant, but I did have her explanation of what was going on, how they needed me, and what I could do to help. I was unprepared for what greeted me when I arrived.

I walked into the room and Alex welcomed me. She looked "okay" but exhausted. Her mom and dad sat at her bedside looking pensive and nurses moved in and about doing the things nurses do. Moments later Alex began to thrash her right arm so violently that it would strike her head unless someone restrained her. Her leg and arm hit the bed with such force that the bed shook and the thrashing was audible from across the room. It became my task to do the restraining so she wouldn't harm herself or any bystanders. We took turns doing this for long periods. It tired us but, more than anything, it seemed impossible for a child to endure this for any length of time. After many of these episodes, Alex began to dislocate her shoulder and her wrist. All of us tried to help relocate her limbs when asked. My specialty became relocating her shoulder. I got so good at it that Alex preferred me to do it, or at least help her to do it. She relocated her wrist herself most of the time. As the severity and rate at which these "spasms" continued, it became evident that this could not go on indefinitely. We continued the restraint process for what seemed like much too long. We all became exhausted in this 24/7 undertaking. This was hard! How could a child continue this way? I felt helpless to assist. It was a low point for me. There were to be many more over the next several weeks.

After Alex's stroke, we kept a vigil at Alex's side continuously at Juli's insistence. I wasn't sure it was necessary at the time. I am now certain that it had a very substantial effect on Alex's recovery rate and was much more important to the extent of her recovery.

Alex remained in a coma for some time. This was to allow the brain swelling to go down. Her medications were gradually lowered until she began coming out of it, a period of several weeks. We read to her, sang to her, and played Enya constantly. If I never hear that music again it will be too soon. I am basically a very optimistic person. I can very nearly always find a way to find the "glass half full," but I was not so certain that my optimism was justified. It was tough to maintain the image, but I did because I believed it important for the others and myself. During this entire period physicians, nurses, residents, and technicians made visits to Alex on a regular basis. In addition they all made a simultaneous visit to her bedside to discuss her case. The family was included in these "rounds" each morning and encouraged to ask questions. Juli took the lead and, when she encouraged the rest of us, we participated as well. The result of this process was that often the questions about the reasons for particular treatment decisions had to be thought through with great care. They permitted everyone to be able to explain the basis for every part of the treatment plan, usually resulting in substantial improvements in the logic and hopefully of the outcomes.

Juli will not accept less from anyone connected with Alex than she believes Alex requires, including Alex. This is not lost on Alex herself; she continuously astonishes me with regard to how hard and how long she is willing to work at what we all believe will make recovery quicker and better, not just once in a while but almost constantly. She developed a spunky attitude like her mom, sister, aunt, and grandma. It is sometimes hard to deal with, but on the whole, essential to progress.

This was a difficult time with so many instances when I felt like I was being hit by a locomotive. However, I was glad to be there to provide whatever help was deemed necessary. I had not been away from Joy for more than a few days in more than fifty years, and that was while I was on active duty with the air force. It was hard on both of us. At least now we had cell phones and conversations didn't require rolls of quarters to complete a long-distance call.

Eventually it was time to return to Florida. Alex continues to do well. This amazing child, with tremendous assistance from her mom, is almost back to being a regular teenager.

Marc's Point of View

My family is strong, stronger than I imagined. I was surprised by the strength of Alex's will to live; before the accident she had a tendency to give into her sickness. Looking back on the steady decline of her health, the unimaginable amount of physical pain she had to endure, the spasms and dislocations, as well as the psychological doubts that the doctors and—it's sad to say—her parents, family, and friends inflicted on her; she overcame and turned out to be my hero. I truly believe that I could not have lived through what she suffered, and I contribute her inner desire to rehabilitate herself while maintaining an exceptionally positive attitude, which mysteriously seemed to appear when she needed it the most, the reason she is with us today, functioning two years into her recovery as a silly semi-independent teenager.

My other daughter, Jessica, should have emotionally collapsed under the long-term family stress and lack of attention.

I constantly worried that even though she is very bright, her OCD and anxieties coupled with our inability to provide the support and attention she seemed to require would cause her to become dysfunctional. We continually passed her to other family and friends while we attended to Alex's numerous emergencies, many times with no notice and for extended periods of time. I underestimated her strength. She not only rose to the occasion, but she handled life and our stress far better than I did. Jessica's resulting emotional wounds are real, and she continues to get hurt by family and friends that only ask how Alex is doing, or only pay "real" attention to Alex's rehabilitation. I recognize that Jessica has a ghost syndrome when Alex is close by. Juli and I tried to help her by sending her to activities where people know only her and not Alex, which did help a little.

It is hard on Jessica, and she feels guilty for those feelings; we all know there is no easy solution, but it is one that she will have to live with for a long time. Jessica knows that Alex is not responsible for how other people act and she tries not to let her anger be directed at Alex; I believe she is successful at that. She is an amazing little big sister—I added the word big because she truly became the big sister to Alex after the stroke, in all areas from Alex's care to recovery.

Jessica has played a key role in helping her sister progress, a role an adult could not fi ll. Jessica's sibling interactions with Alex, from playing to sisterly arguing, stimulated Alex's brain. They were best friends before the illness and have remained close through Alex's changes, which was not easy and usually more on the difficult side. Since Alex's stroke and personality shift, she has a tendency to constantly mother Jessica, and having two mothers is not easy. Eventually Jessica attended the same middle school as Alex and Jessica felt nervous about it. Alex is so much more spontaneous than she was before the stroke. Jessica is more on the reserved side and worries about the attention she gets from being Alex's sister. If I had to elect the best sister in the world award, I think Jessica would be a top candidate for all she has done for Alex, all she has had to put up with due to Alex, and all the love she has for her family. She is amazing.

Juli is an educated, logical, smart, strong woman with a lot of common sense. I believe she played the key role in saving Alex's life and helping Alex to recover as well as she has. Juli is competitive and never gives up. I believe that many people think they understand what it is like not to give up, but I have rarely seen anyone be so competitive. This competitiveness and never-giving-up attitude was ultimately tested by Alex and all I can say is that at times it is all Juli had to rely on, or should I say all *we* had left to rely on. I will never forget the time when it looked bleak and Juli lectured the hospital staff to have hope; it helped focus everyone's attitude. Juli also had strong beliefs that Alex needed to know we were not only in the room, but that a family member was awake and by her side twenty-four hours a day, seven days a week. We read books to her, talked to her, touched her, and played soothing music over and over and over . . . .

I believe a person in a coma or coming out of a coma may be at times slightly aware of noises, voices, words that go on around them, but they are unable to respond or are too slow to respond. Talking to Alex shortly after she gained her ability to communicate with us, I was led to believe that there were times when she sensed we were with her. I think Juli's early idea to reach out to Alex was one of many great ideas she had for us to help Alex come back to us. Another important strength Juli had was to recognize Alex's situation and feelings and to constantly remind me of how Alex must feel, giving me a perspective on Alex's point of view or situation, instead of how I felt during each situation or calamity. This did not come naturally to me, and her words allowed me to better direct my actions in order to become a better father. I could go on forever about all the special things Juli is capable of and how they made a difference, but I will end by saying that Juli is a natural teacher and parent. She approaches teaching and parenting from every angle imaginable; even though she and I made mistakes, she was able to recognize when necessary changes needed to be made and implemented our course corrections for Alex's best interest.

Examining myself, I find that Alex's long illness affected me to my core, forever changing my understanding of how delicate the mind is, including our personalities and sanity. I saw and dealt with the widest range of emotions, sometimes in the same day. The psychological effects of the illness, of pain, not understanding, doubts, prescription drugs, lack of sleep, and so on all surprised me. I made a decision, no matter how bad it got, not to take any medication or substance to help me handle this terrible situation. No matter how bad I felt, my family needed 100 percent of me for support and decisions. I battled depression and deep sadness to the point where even good memories or family photos hurt to think about or see. I was tested as a person and father, and I know that I did my very best to help Alex, Jessica, and Juli. I also recognize that I made mistakes, ones I wish I could take back.

I feel fortunate to have had Dr. Alden as my daughter's doctor. I wish there were more people like him in this world. He listened and truly cared on a deep personal level; he is a special person, with charisma and stature. I think about him and his wife often and wish I had a way to show him how much I appreciated his help.

Now that it has been two years since Alex's stroke and amazing recovery, I still possess strong mixed emotions. I feel fortunate that Alex has reached a level where she is an active member and participant of our family and sad over her being a different person, one who will not have the same potential she once had. It is still early and we provide the absolute best rehabilitation for her, so we do not know how far she will actually recover. I am grateful for what our family has. Now I better understand others' pain and misfortune. I also never thought my family could reach a point of feeling normal, but it pleasantly happens more often now. I guess we are all healing and beginning to move on.

Alex's Perspective

Sometimes people have things going on in their lives. Sometimes people feel pain, suffering, and sorrow. And sometimes people just want to give up. But even if you are getting worse, you can never give up.

I felt all of those feelings. Sometimes I felt like just giving up myself, but if I gave up I never would have become what I am today and I never would have succeeded. I learned that you can never give up. I learned that working hard pays off. And, I learned that you have to laugh a little.

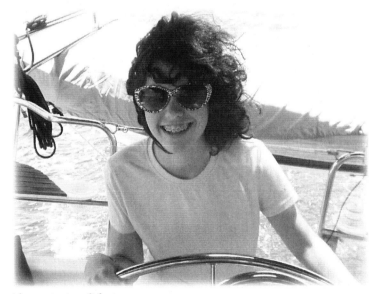

Alex enjoying life.

Two Chances

Life is a gift,
Don't use it up.

You could keep going
And never look back.

Or you could stay for a while
And look back to your past.

You can succeed
if you put your mind to it.

Trying is believing
and believing is trying.

Life is a miracle, a challenge no less.
A challenge is a hard thing to bear.

My mom always says, "Try once and if you don't succeed try, try again,"
And I live by that motto.

Life is like a bowl of soup. Sometimes it's hot and it
burns you.
Sometimes it's cold and you feel a little bit
lonesome.

A memory can walk with you for the rest of your life,
Some good memories and some bad.

A memory is the most valuable thing you can have,
So think about it.

But don't forget life IS a gift
You need to be thankful!

—By Alex Dixon (age 14), April 2012

EPILOGUE

Three years have passed since Alex's stroke. She is more than halfway through her freshman year of high school. Her transformation has been amazing. This year was her first year going to school full-time. She is in all regular classes, although she still needs a full-time one-on-one aide. She has almost straight A's. She studies all the time. She takes the regular school bus to and from school every day and spends every afternoon and evening and each weekend studying. She does not read well enough yet to read to learn and so we read her textbooks to her each night. We review everything she learns at school every evening. She continues to learn to read and she practices writing whenever she can. Everything just takes so long. It takes her about forty-five minutes to write one paragraph. What would take a normal high school freshman one hour to complete takes Alex four. With all her efforts, I would estimate her reading to be on a fifth-grade level and her writing to be just above that. Her comprehension is sometimes much higher and her fluency much lower. Her math is on grade level with some gaps here and there. For example, when we get to percents and I tell her to think of percent as per one hundred because there are 100 cents in a dollar, she just looks at me with a confused expression. It is then that I realize I have yet to reteach her coins and their values.

With all the support we have been resolute about putting in place, such as the extra help with schoolwork at home and special services in school, she is getting there. Her aide takes notes for her in school so she can focus on the teacher. Her aide also records what occurs in class and what homework Alex needs to complete in a notebook for me so I can help Alex stay on top of her assignments and keep up with her peers. This is not something she can do independently at this point, although she is taking on more responsibility than in previous years. She is able to begin some of her homework on her own where she was not able to do so before.

We believe she will graduate from high school but we assume that it will take tremendous effort all four years, including summers. From there she plans to attend a community college and then a university—not bad for a cucumber. High school will likely be the most challenging part of the journey. In college she can go at her own pace and focus on fewer subjects. High school seems to have far more requirements to be completed in such a limited amount of time. The time is limited because she is determined to graduate with her peers rather than take longer. We don't yet know where Alex will attend college. I hope she will attend in our hometown but that might not be my decision. I'm sure she will make wherever she goes her home. She is so sweet to all she meets.

Alex has a few friends in school who have stuck by her side. There are some who have not; they haven't been mean to her— they've just moved on. That might have occurred under normal circumstances but we will never know. Those that have stuck with her watch out for her; they paint her nails and do her hair. They find ways to interact with Alex on her terms although she is often quite intent about protecting them, as well, and watching out for their feelings. Alex loves to shop for her friends, buying thoughtful gifts that are full of meaning. In school people are kind to her and greet her throughout the day. She still has some trouble remembering their names. She is getting better at conversations with peers but it still takes effort. Most everything takes effort.

She no longer attends formal therapy. She was released from those at the beginning of last summer, against our will as usual. That left us in a position to begin "DIY" therapy, or do-it-yourself therapy. I think we've done pretty well.

DIY therapy has required some serious creativity on our part. We use everything at our disposal and then some. Alex relearned to swim and now she swims laps in our pool whenever weather permits. Early in Alex's illness we discussed with one of her physical therapists what a good therapy pool might include. We had a pool designed and built in our backyard that included most of those suggestions. It is shallow and long but also has places that are beyond where Alex can stand so she can work on treading water or wear a float around her waist and do exercises. We try to find therapeutic value in pretty much all of our activities. At first glance, our home seems full of fun games and they *are* fun, but when you probe more deeply you learn that almost everything has a therapeutic purpose.

We went online to find used games we could use for therapy. We bought a huge air hockey table. We use that to help Alex with left hand-eye coordination. She pretty much beats everyone who dares to play against her these days. We also bought a foosball table. At first she made anyone who played her use his or her less dominant hand only, but that is no longer necessary. She beats me now when I am playing with both hands.

We purchased any game we could think of that might improve her vocabulary and general speech. One of our favorites is HEDBANZ™ by Spin Master. This game is played with each player wearing a plastic headband with a card stuck to the front of it facing out, so your opponents can see it but you cannot. A card might read, "I am a hamburger," and have a picture of a hamburger under the words. The object is to ask your opponents yes or no questions until you accumulate enough clues to guess your card. It is a pretty funny game, made even more hilarious when played with a participant who has aphasia. Alex is a great sport when playing this game and I think it has provided a fun way for her to focus on speech therapy. She also likes the Scrabble game SLAM! by Parker Brothers. This game is intended to be a fast-paced word game where four-letter words are made by replacing just one letter of the previous four-letter word. We change the rules as we do with most games we play so that time is not a factor in the game. We take turns changing the word so that Alex has the "think time" she needs to be successful. On games like Blokus^R by Mattel, Alex needs no extra time. She is a competitor whether we use extended time or not. She is quite good with spatial-strategy games, reminding me that not all of her brain is damaged.

I've noticed that we've begun to play fewer games these days. Alex still asks to play them but I often say we don't have time. Balancing all that needs to occur with fun is a real challenge. I have to remind myself of the importance of being silly more often now. I can feel myself slip into a rut of nagging more often than before and I don't like it. When I begin to feel that way, Marc often suggests that Alex and I go for a bike ride before continuing with our studies. Those bike rides do wonders for my attitude and interactions with Alex. Really, Alex has done wonders for me as a human being. I am a better person because of my interactions with her and I am not alone with these feelings. Just one bike ride and I am back on this better path.

We bought an adult-size tricycle and strapped Alex's right foot to the pedal. We moved the hand break to the left handle bar so she could control it and off she went. In the beginning, her right foot would get stuck in the pedal every few rotations. We tried everything to keep it in place. We used large rubber bands, ace bandages, and duct tape. Marc or I walked next to her and readjusted her foot over and over again. Eventually, we found a better way to attach her foot using a modified toe cage and her leg got stronger. Now her foot rarely gets stuck. She rides so fast we can no longer walk alongside her; rather we bike with her. We even had gears added to her tricycle so she can go faster and farther. We try to ride our neighborhood a few times per week; it is about a three and a half mile loop. At one point last summer Alex got bored with the same path so we decided to try something new.

I pushed, pulled, grunted, and heaved until I got Alex's forty-five-pound tricycle into the back of my minivan and strapped my bike on the rack in back. Jessica was away at camp and Marc was at work, so it was just Alex and me. We drove to a paved bike trail and set off on our excursion. It was short-lived. The paved path wasn't very wide. Alex rode in front of me in the center of the path. Before long some kids came upon us riding their bikes from the other direction. I said, "Alex, move over a little. Okay, that's enough. Alex, hit the brake, hit the brake, hit the brake!" She moved over and just kept going, right off the edge of the path and down a five-foot ditch. She never slowed down. She couldn't see it. She cannot see to the right. Her foot was strapped to the pedal so her forty-five-pound tricycle landed on top of her. I thought I broke her neck. I jumped off my bike and scrambled down after her. The ditch had a sheer drop with vines growing up along the sides. I yanked the tricycle off of her and threw it to the side. I have no idea where the strength to do that came from. As luck would have it, she landed in an ant pile. They were not red ants and did not bite but I didn't know it at the time. I screamed for her to climb out of the ditch. She couldn't make any headway with the vines. She lost her shoe in her efforts to get out. I climbed up in front of her and grabbed her under her armpits and dragged her out of the ditch. I carried her to the middle of the bike path, stood her up, and slapped all the ants off of her while she just stood there stunned and covered in dirt. Once I dragged her tricycle out of the ditch, I made her get back on and keep going. She was not happy about it but she knew I was right to make her get back on. However, we both knew that Marc was going to have a fit when he found out. He tends to think I push too hard and risk a little too much. I was not looking forward to sharing this latest incident with him. When we got back to the car, Alex got on her cell phone and called everyone she could think of to tell them her mother drove her off a cliff—including Marc. That's my girl. Now whenever someone experiences difficulties and wants to quit, she tells them they have to get back on the bike like she had to and it works.

The tricycle helps with strength and endurance but not with balance. We use a paddleboard for that. We began with Alex sitting in front of me and me paddling along the Intracoastal Waterway. Neither of us had ever been on a paddleboard before last summer. Our first few outings were pretty funny. First I had to get from the dock to the paddleboard, then I had to lift Alex onto the paddleboard. We rocked and hooted but we both made it on. At first it was enough for Alex to balance while sitting in front of me, with me standing and paddling. Eventually I wanted her to stand, but she was frightened; she didn't think she was ready but I knew she was. Ultimately, it took me lifting her up by the shoulders of her lifejacket to get her standing. Once she stood she was hooked. She would stand for very short periods on each outing. Now Alex paddles for part of every trip. I stand behind her to help when she needs it and to give her breaks so she can sit while I paddle. Sometimes we take out a two-man kayak instead. She has paddled by manatees and dolphins. We have fallen off and climbed back on. It is our favorite form of "therapy."

Alex is determined to find a sport in addition to paddleboarding. She takes tennis lessons occasionally. She plays to the best of her ability but it is pretty funny. Her run is a bit strange, and she plays with her left hand, of course. When she tries to start a ball and drop it from her right hand, she cannot get her hand to release it. She stands there shaking her hand until the ball falls out and she can swing at it. The worst part is her vision; because she cannot see to the right, the ball pegs her frequently—she doesn't see it coming. We laugh pretty hard during tennis. Laughter is still our best strategy for almost everything we do.

Other therapy takes the form of life skills. I read somewhere that therapy is most successful when the task is completed for a greater purpose. For example, Alex makes her bed most mornings with her right hand. Her bed is pretty messy but the goal of making her bed might help Alex to engage her hand more readily than just placing pegs in pegboards and then taking them back out again. She is focused on completing a task. She clears part of the table with her right hand—only the things that are not breakable. Her hand is still her weakest link but she has not given up. She is back to playing the piano. My mother found a piano book for left-handed piano and Alex can now play those pieces very well. However, she also tries to play with her right hand. Those pieces touch my heart more.

What also touches my heart are Alex's efforts taking American Sign Language (ASL). That knowledge never came back to her after her stroke so she enrolled in ASL in high school. She tries to sign with both hands. She is getting easier to understand. She is often surprised when she videotapes herself signing because in her mind she sees herself signing equally with both hands. I hope she keeps seeing herself that way. I hope even more that she can return to that.

It is interesting how the way Alex sees herself has evolved. After the stroke she was the epitome of optimism and motivation; she didn't seem to compare herself to her pre-stroke self. She was happy with her accomplishments and truly proud of all she did. As time has passed, we've seen a bit of a shift. Alex has become a bit sad about what she's lost. At times she says that she wishes her right hand worked so she could play the piano the way she used to play. She says that it is frustrating and embarrassing to struggle with reading when she knows she used to read so well. She is worried that when students in school hear her read they think she is not smart.

Just recently, Alex was assigned a career project in freshman English. She was required to take an interest survey and a basic skills survey. The results of those surveys determined a set of careers from which she needed to make a selection to research. Marc and I were very worried about this project. At that point, Alex was still telling all she knew that she planned to be a neurologist. While not out of the question, Marc and I have come to think that this career path is unlikely. We know how much support she needs now to succeed in standard classes in ninth grade. We are exhausted and are not sure how we can keep up this pace of support through medical school. We will if she needs us but I would be remiss if I didn't say we don't worry about it. Alex chose neurology because she wanted to prevent other children from being treated like she had been. The career exercise helped her to realize that she might be more well-suited for child life specialist. We are thrilled with this shift. Alex will still help children but she will do so through her strengths. Still, the project was not easy as it caused Alex to realize more of her weaknesses. At these times we find it necessary to get psychological boosts from her psychologist, Dr. Stewart. He continues to be an important part of Alex's village. He can reinstate her "Yes I Can" attitude faster than anyone else.

Alex's village has shifted. She is beginning to move out of the center of attention more and more and that is good. Her focus is more on helping others than on herself. She gets less special treatment at school and she is learning to manage. I do think that without her aide this would not be as positive. Even so there are bumps. At midyear Alex went into chorus as an elective. She was thrilled to take a class that might place her on equal footing with her peers. She was excited right up until the class started and she realized that many of the songs they sang were in other languages. She said, "Mom, I can barely read English, how am I going to do this?" I said, "Just like you do everything else: to the best of your ability." She kept that attitude when a choreographer included dance with the songs for the spring concert.

Alex wants to help people and to ensure that students with special needs have the opportunity to live their best lives. To that end, she recently gave a talk for education majors at my university. Her talk was entitled "Waiting on the world to change: A student with special needs shares her story and suggestions for change." During her presentation, Alex shared how she felt when she first got sick, that there was nothing worse in this world, that life wasn't worth living. Then she shared how she felt after the stroke: that she was lucky to be alive, that she could accomplish anything if she worked hard enough. She discussed how, when teachers believe in her and help her to be a contributing member in class, she feels accepted and complete, but that when teachers don't work to make connections she feels lost and frustrated. She shared funny stories and sad stories. The forty participants went from laughing to crying to laughing again. Alex was so comfortable in this arena, helping teachers to meet the needs of all learners. As I watched Alex, I saw a young woman who is comfortable in her skin and who helps others to feel comfortable around her while simultaneously discussing important, and often uncomfortable, issues. Alex will create change. She will move mountains as she shares her message of hope, determination, and strategies to support those in need.

Alex continues to pull us along through song and by example. One of her more recent theme songs is "My Wish." My wish for Alex is that she can enjoy a complete recovery, but she is scarred—scarred by doctors who didn't believe her.

She has been having some trouble with the wire to her deep brain stimulator recently. It is not uncoiling as she grows and it is beginning to pull the battery in her chest up toward her neck. We made an appointment with a neurosurgeon to explore options but we could not get an appointment immediately. I was running on my treadmill one morning—still trying to lose the weight I gained during this ordeal—when I got a call from Alex on my cell phone. She was calling me from school and she was crying hysterically.

She said, "What if they don't believe me? What if they think I'm faking?"

I said, "Alex, they can see that the battery is being pulled just by looking at you."

"But Mom, they could see that my foot was twisted too and they didn't believe me."

"Alex, don't let those people who didn't believe in you win. You must continue to believe in yourself or they win."

She understood, calmed down, and returned to class.

I stood on my treadmill with sweat pouring down my back and tears streaming down my face. She is so strong and yet so fragile. While this is a description of Alex, it is also a description of me—I think I just might hide it better. I wrote this book about

Alex—it was her stroke of luck—but I am left thinking how it really is a head fake like Randy Pausch's *The Last Lecture*. He wrote a book about achieving his childhood dreams prior to his death but in the lecture that inspired the book he tells the audience that it is really a head fake. The lecture isn't for the audience; it is for his children so they will learn more about their dad and they will know to live their best lives. Is *A Stroke of Luck* about Alex or is it about me? Have I used the path of Alex's journey to make sense of my own experiences and ultimate growth? Maybe. It really doesn't matter; in many ways we are inextricably connected for now, but not forever. She will grow up and continue to forge her path independently. How she will make her way through this world remains to be seen.

I turn my iPod back on and continue my run. The next song on my playlist is another one of Alex's songs, "Beautiful" by Christina Aguilera. I am reminded of Alex's inner strength and beauty—no matter what they say.

She will make it because she was given a second chance at life—and she took it.

Acknowledgments

In order to acknowledge people for making this book possible, I need to begin by thanking those who helped Alex to survive this ordeal. For this I am obviously appreciative beyond what words could ever describe.

My first thanks go to my husband, Marc Dixon. We were a team as we searched for answers, cures, even the right questions to ask. He is very strong. He is strong in his commitment to do what is right, in his support for my efforts, and in his love for our family. I continue to depend on that strength.

I thank my co-author and younger daughter, Jessica, whose cerebral approach to living allowed her to examine her life as she knew it while it unfolded around her and used writing to help her put it back together.

My parents, Joy and Harvey Inventasch, put their lives on hold while Alex was sick to be where we needed when we needed, sometimes when we didn't even know we needed them. They continue to do so. They are an integral part of Alex's recovery. The process of writing this book opened wounds created by being a part of Alex's struggle with her illness that had barely healed for them, yet they were supportive throughout.

Really, all my and Marc's family have been there for us in so many ways throughout this ordeal. Marni, Valerie, Sherri, David, Gary, Tara, Bruce, JoAnn, Grannie (Vergie), Eileen, Ron, Bob, and Charlanne contributed at points and, more often, throughout this journey.

Many of my friends played significant roles in supporting me as I struggled to find ways to help Alex. My thanks go to Ed Nolan, Lisa Dieker, Thomasenia Adams, Aurora Richards, Frances Grinstead, Sherron Roberts, Janet Andreasen, and Rayna Yaker. Alex's support team included her caregivers and aids. Thank you to Ms. Sue Bresnahan, Miss Norie, Michelle Robinson, Jessica Weber, and Kathy Murphy, in particular, but to so many others as well. Also, thanks go to Alex's teachers—who worked so hard to help her succeed, especially Ms. Poarch, Ms. Capp, Dr. Stephan, Ms. Carpenter, and so many more. To Alex's village—thanks for being my village too.

It really took a village to handle what we encountered both medically and emotionally. So many doctors, nurses, psychologists, occupational therapists, physical therapists, and speech therapists were tireless in their efforts to help Alex. I am thankful for whatever parts they played in Alex's road to recovery. I am especially thankful for Alex's pediatrician ("Dr. Conway"), Alex's psychologist (Dr. Stewart), and Alex's neurosurgeon ("Dr. Alden").

As Alex's recovery seemed possible, I started to share her story with teachers across the country during my professional speaking engagements. Upon hearing her story, they encouraged me to share it with others. I'm not sure I could have gone through with this project without their support.

My own colleagues were so supportive. My boss, Dr. Mike Hynes, protected me from myself and allowed me to thrive when many would have left their profession even though they loved what they did. My colleagues in mathematics education stepped in to teach my classes, providing my students with consistency and an excellent education. My graduate students understood why I was overwhelmed at times, but still knew that I would give it my all—I am thankful for their patience in allowing me to do so.

Writing this book was a much bigger project than what I first imagined. I had written several mathematics books but I had no idea what went into a book like this. So many people reviewed the book, giving me useful feedback and encouragement—I am thankful to all of them for the unique perspectives they provided. I found Lisa Tener one afternoon as I searched the web for ideas and support—I was close to giving up on the idea of writing Alex's story. I responded to her blog with a question about this book. It was the first time I ever contributed to a blog. She responded within a day. She offered to read my book. I was back on track. She provided very helpful feedback and eventually introduced me to Stuart Horwitz. Stuart's Book Architecture Method helped me to see what I meant to write before I ever wrote it. His critiques were to the point, significant at times, and always laced with humor, making them easier to handle and address. When it looked like I might publish the book, he and Chloe Marsala helped me to make the idea of telling Alex's story in print a reality. I am so thankful for this.

Jordan Barrett is a dear, long-time family friend. Marc knows him as Uncle Jordy. When it was time to design the cover of the book, Marc called him for advice. Jordy asked to read the book and created a cover that at once displayed Alex's journey and hope for continued recovery. He described in one picture what it took me far, far more than a thousand words to write.

Above all, I am most thankful to Alex for allowing me to tell her story. Many of the pages of this book describe scenes she was in but only learned about through hearing this story. These pages include topics and experiences that are very personal. Alex agreed to open up her life for others to read because she wants to help people. I am so very thankful to Alex just for being Alex and for being with us.

About the Authors

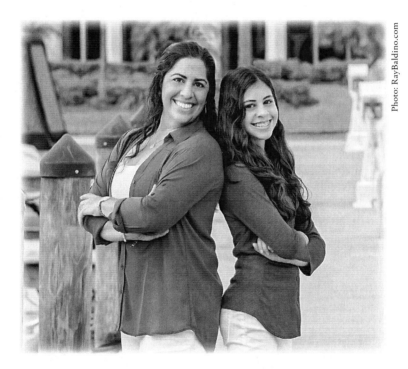

Photo: RayBaldino.com

Juli K. Dixon, Ph.D. is a professor of mathematics education at the University of Central Florida (UCF). She coordinates the award-winning Lockheed Martin/UCF Academy Master of Education in K-8 Mathematics and Science and the Ph.D. in Mathematics Education. She is a prolific writer who has published books, textbooks, book chapters, and articles. A sought-after speaker, Dr. Dixon has delivered keynotes and other presentations throughout the United States. She has served as chair of the National Council of Teachers of Mathematics Student Explorations in Mathematics Editorial Panel and as a member of the Association of Mathematics Teacher Educators, the Nevada Mathematics Council, and the Florida Association of Mathematics Teacher Educators Boards of Directors.

Jessica Dixon began writing this book when she was eleven years old. She completed her last chapter just after she turned thirteen. She enjoys reading, writing poetry, sailing, kayaking, rock climbing, playing tennis, and playing the French horn. She has already achieved success in competitions with her Odyssey of the Mind team and for her National History Day project—making it to the state level with each. She is contemplating what she wants to "be" when she grows up, and she is seeing that her choices are wide open.